# BABY
# WEIGHT

## The Complete Guide to Prenatal & Postpartum Fitness

Micky Marie Morrison, PT, ICPFE

ISBN #978-0615522586

Photographs by Santiago Albert Pons
albertpons.com

Author photograph by Agustina Bombardó

Illustrations by Juan Pablo Canale Banus
canalebanus. com

Cover and book design by Brad Eller
bradeller.com

Printed in the United States of America

Body Works Media
87200 Overseas Hwy. Suite A-10
Islamorada, FL 33036

babyweightfitness.com

Dedicated to the Fabulous Burga Boys: Bernardo, Makani, and my love, Javier.

Your support and understanding made this book possible. Your love makes life worth living.

# Acknowledgements

This book wouldn't have been possible without the support of a tribe of expecting and new mothers, friends, family, teachers, and colleagues.

First, I must thank my parents, Sherry Lynn Brobeck and Don Morrison for giving me the tenacity and belief in myself to carry this project to completion.

I am eternally grateful to my devoted husband, Javier Burga, whose enthusiasm was sometimes greater than mine for this book. Your belief in me gives me strength and helps me find the best of myself to give.

A million thanks, and more, to my dearest friends Jon and Wanda Headrick, whose lifetime of love and support has been a stabilizing force that changed my life's course.

Thank you, Bernardo and Makani, for forgoing playtime so that mommy could write in the last few months of finishing this book.

Thanks so much to the CoreMamas™ and their babies, for their dedication to the classes and their patience with the long photo shoots: Joanna Lardizabal and Sabrina, Katie Cunningham Pokorny and Santiago, Lucy Ashman and Orrin, Marissa Shefveland and Norma Angelina, Cindy Phillips and Lindsey, Machteld Oosterban and Diago, and Shannon Dewald and Zoe.

A big thank you goes to my dear friend Cindy Lech, whose kind words and unwavering friendship were instrumental in this and many previous accomplishments.

I am grateful to my friend Christine K. Wilson, for sharing in the book-making drama with me, and pushing me to get it finished.

I cannot thank enough Dr. Leighanne Glazener for her reading and revising, advising, and encouraging.

Thanks also to Dr. Carlos Botas for taking the time to read the book, and for liking it!

Thank you Dr. Luis Sanjose for treating childbirth like a natural miracle rather than a medical procedure and for making my own birth experience amazing and gratifying.

Thanks to the patient and dedicated designer Brad Eller, and to the reluctant but brilliant photographer Santiago Albert Pons. Your vision helped make this book beautiful.

A very special thanks goes out to a very special woman, Patricia McNair, whose strong character, feistiness, and love for words made her a valuable resource as well as a cherished friend, and whose constant inquisitiveness helped push me to finish.

# Contents

# Foreword

What an amazing time of life! There is no point when your body will undergo more rapid changes and physical challenges than during pregnancy, childbirth and the postpartum period. While exciting, this is also stressful, and you probably have some concerns about coping with it all. *Baby Weight* has the answers.

With over 20 years of experience as an obstetrician, I am convinced a physically fit woman has a better pregnancy outcome. She is less likely to suffer from complications of pregnancy such as hypertension and gestational diabetes, she is better equipped to deal with the rigors of labor and postpartum recovery and her chances for cesarean section are lower. As a bonus, she recovers her postpartum shape more quickly.

In *Baby Weight,* Micky Morrison presents a simple, sensible plan to help you avoid excessive weight gain and maintain healthy muscle tone during pregnancy, and to recover your form quickly after giving birth. The nutritional advice is practical, effective and easy to implement. Micky's experience as a physical therapist adds a dimension that other perinatal fitness books and exercise plans lack. Micky responsibly addresses issues such as pelvic floor dysfunction and diastasis recti to help women avoid future complications, and teaches women how to prevent or alleviate common aches and pains through exercise. With a professional understanding of the special needs of the pregnant and postpartum woman, Micky developed safe and effective exercises that are more challenging than the usual prenatal or postpartum program. Special modifications to the exercises allow women who have had a cesarean to safely begin exercise after surgery. The postpartum program teaches you to exercise with your baby so you can spend quality time together while you work out.

Whether you have recently given birth and are looking for a way to get back your "pre-baby" shape, or you are early in your pregnancy and hoping to minimize the impact on your body, *Baby Weight* offers tools to reach your fitness goals. You will learn how to eat during and after pregnancy to manage your weight, and how to exercise safely and effectively to achieve and maintain muscle tone.

Keep reading, take some *action* and you'll be on your way to a healthier, happier pregnancy and recovery!

*Leighanne Glazener, M.D., F.A.C.O.G*

# Author's Note

## THE BIRTH OF BABY WEIGHT

In my 15 years of experience as a women's health physical therapist, I have treated many mothers. A significant percentage of those mothers sought treatment for conditions resulting from their inability to recover muscle tone and strength lost during pregnancy and childbirth and to lose the weight gained during pregnancy. The most common contributing factor found among them was a general lack of knowledge of how to lose the weight and get fit. Even those who made their best efforts were often unsuccessful because they unknowingly sabotaged their diets, and the exercise they chose didn't effectively isolate the weak spots, allowing them to compensate with stronger muscle groups. The resulting complications varied from chronic low back pain, neck and shoulder pain, pelvic floor dysfunction, and abdominal muscle separation, to obesity and general deconditioning, and in some cases persisted for years after giving birth.

Having seen first-hand how a woman's baby weight can negatively impact her life, it was no wonder that when I found myself pregnant at age 30, I was terrified that I would gain 50 or 60 pounds and have a hard time losing it. I took action by extensively researching nutrition and safe exercise practices during pregnancy and obtained certification through the International Childbirth Education Association as a perinatal fitness educator. I created a diet plan based on healthy nutritional choices with daily indulgences to avoid feeling deprived. Despite the fact that I was the girl who gained 23 rather than the usual 15 pounds in the first semester of college, I was able to control my weight gain during pregnancy and keep it in the healthy range at an absolutely average 26 pounds.

My training as a physical therapist gave me the insight to challenge conservative medical views about exercise during pregnancy. My supportive obstetrician encouraged me to continue to teach an abdominal toning class at the local gym until the eighth month of my pregnancy. In modifying various exercises for myself as the pregnancy progressed, I developed a program of safe and super-effective core exercises that my non-pregnant students loved, which I would later call the CoreMama™ program. During the first weeks after giving birth, I began to do the same exercises, with a twist – I did them *with* my baby. I realized I didn't have to go to the gym, or get dressed, or find a sitter and leave my precious and demanding newborn on the sidelines to start getting back into shape. That is when "baby weight" began to mean something entirely different to me. And soon it will for you, too.

Micky Marie Morrison, PT, ICPFE

# Introduction

## Baby Weight: Your Prenatal and Postpartum Fitness Plan

Get your body back faster by using your baby's weight to help you lose your baby weight! The *Baby Weight* Fitness Plan provides a comprehensive wellness strategy for expectant and new mothers to help manage their baby weight, beginning with a practical nutrition plan to guide food choices during and after pregnancy. You will learn how to incorporate a healthy diet and regular exercise into your daily routine to make it part of your lifestyle rather than a chore. *Baby Weight* combines a variety of everyday cardiovascular training activities with the CoreMama™ exercises that teach you to isolate the exact muscles weakened during pregnancy and childbirth so that you tone all the right spots and burn the calories needed to reduce the extra weight gained during pregnancy.

## Be a CoreMama™, Fit to the Core

The CoreMama™ program includes prenatal exercises to help expectant mothers get and stay in shape before the big event by training the specific muscles of childbirth and those involved in a speedy postnatal recovery. What sets the CoreMama™ program apart from others is the intensity of the workout gained through very low impact exercises that isolate the muscles that need the most work. You will sweat; you will tremble, and you will definitely feel like you have had a workout when you are finished with the exercises.

Once your baby is born, the postnatal exercises in the CoreMama™ program will allow you to use the resistance of your baby's weight to regain strength in the core muscle groups weakened during pregnancy. These exercises are specifically designed to help you lose unwanted inches and pounds. The positioning and handling techniques, derived from my experience as a neonatal and pediatric physical therapist, help stimulate your baby's gross motor development while integrating her* into the exercises. The CoreMama™ program's unique approach to postpartum exercise promotes bonding with your baby while you grow stronger together. Even a new mother can find at least 15 minutes a day to interact with her baby with these low impact but intense exercises that are fun for both you and your baby. The added resistance of your baby's weight helps maximize the effects of the exercises.

Since developing the CoreMama™ exercises, I have had the joy of teaching them to numerous expectant and new mothers with their babies, both in private physical therapy or personal training consultations as well as in group classes. The proof of the program is in the results, which have shown time and again that targeting the muscles weakened during pregnancy can actually make you stronger as your pregnancy progresses. The CoreMama™ program also helps you bounce back to your prenatal shape more quickly and easily after delivery. Without fail, every woman who participated in the program reported looking and feeling better overall.

The psychological benefits of devoting even a few minutes a day to yourself are immense, especially when you can do it guilt-free without leaving your baby. Exercise and bonding with your baby have something in common biologically: both produce endorphins, oxytocin, and other feel-good neurotransmitters that activate the limbic system, the brain's pleasure center. The *Baby Weight* Fitness Plan becomes a good prescription for fighting off the baby blues and for getting back into those favorite blue jeans.

For those who are lucky enough to discover *Baby Weight* before giving birth, you will find the guidance you need to make the right prenatal choices regarding nutrition and exercise to help ensure a satisfying birth experience and a rapid recovery.

For new mothers, you are most likely still coming out of your postpartum daze, finally getting the nerve to pick up this book and to even *think* about getting your body back to its pre-partum state. Don't be disheartened by the sight of your flaccid midsection and the daunting task of recovering your form. Never fear, you have made the first step and are on the right track to feeling better and getting your body back!

*For simplicity's sake and from feminist tendencies, I have chosen to refer to the baby as "she" throughout *Baby Weight*, even though my own babies are both boys.

# The CoreMamas™ and Their Baby Weight Babies

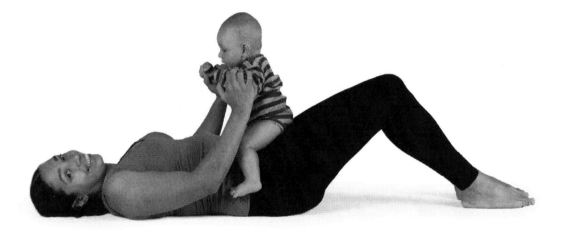

Many thanks to all the *Baby Weight* models. All are real mothers with their own babies who participated in the CoreMama™ classes during and/or after pregnancy.

## LUCY AND ORRIN

Lucy was 36 weeks pregnant for the first photo shoot. She delivered Orrin vaginally without medication and without complication at term. Orrin was 4 months old at the second shoot. Lucy started the CoreMama™ classes 9 months after giving birth to Orrin's older brother, Oliver. About her experience, she says:

"When I started training with Micky about 9 months after my first baby was born, I had been tired, overweight, and out of shape for too long and was finally ready to do something about it. My core muscles were weak and neglected, so I found the classes ·ery difficult at first. I gained strength and confidence quickly, though, and was soon    to do the things I couldn't in the beginning. The classes were tough but I felt great ' them regularly twice a week.

' was pregnant again a few months later, I was able to continue the routine.

a sweat and got a great workout, and even got stronger as my pregnancy progressed. I always left the class feeling more fit and energized, yet relaxed.

I continued to lose the baby weight from my first pregnancy well into the second. Of course, I gained weight during the pregnancy, but while my baby kept growing, and so did my belly, the rest of me got leaner and stronger. On my regular check ups, my docor was amazed a couple of times when I was the same weight as on the previous occasion even though the baby had gained a pound or more. I had actually lost weight! I got bigger, but felt lighter.

Micky pushes us to our max – her favorite mantras are: "Trembling is good" and "It's only by pushing ourselves a little further each time that we grow stronger." Yet she is very conscious of the different needs and abilities of each person, offering various modifications to the exercises. Because she is a physiotherapist, I felt safe doing Micky's exercises until the last week of pregnancy and started back only 2 weeks after Orrin was born.

When I compare the experience of my second pregnancy to the first, the biggest difference is how I felt. I was healthier, stronger, thinner, and better prepared for the new arrival. The labor and delivery were much easier the second time around and I recovered much faster. I definitely thank Micky and CoreMama™ for that."

## JOANNA AND SABRINA

Joanna is Baby Weight's cover girl.  She was 34 weeks pregnant on the back cover, and 4 months postpartum on the front cover.  She delivered Sabrina vaginally without

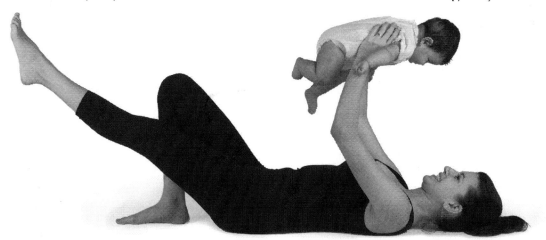

complication at term. Joanna attended the CoreMama™ classes regularly from 17 weeks until 38 weeks pregnant. Here's what she had to say about her experience:

"Micky's classes saved me! I needed direction on how to exercise while I was pregnant, and I found being with other pregnant women in the class motivating and energizing. At first I thought I wouldn't be able to do the exercises, but I got stronger quickly and could do a little more every time. As I got bigger, I was surprised that my belly was not in the way and that I could keep pushing myself to new limits. Micky is a knowledgeable and talented physical therapist. I felt safe to continue challenging myself under her direction. After I had Sabrina, I attended a few classes and continued the exercises at home with my baby. I felt stronger and fitter every day, and we both enjoyed the exercise time together. I am excited Micky is sharing her program with the world now!"

## MARISSA AND ANGELINA

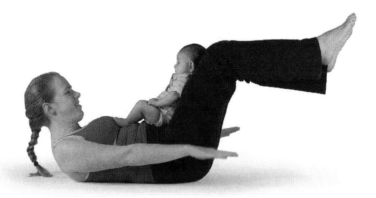

Marissa was 32 weeks pregnant at the time of the first photo shoot, and Angelina was 3 months old at the second shoot. Marissa started the CoreMama™ classes at 27 weeks. She delivered Angelina naturally, without medication and without complication, at term.

"I started participating in Micky's class at the insistence of a coworker who was also pregnant and looking for an exercise buddy. At the time, I wasn't really interested in exercising, but liked the idea of doing something active with other moms-to-be. I worried that the class would be beyond my abilities, but I found the challenge inspiring and began to look forward to the classes. I especially liked that Micky made sure that we did the exercises at our ability level and reminded us to listen to our bodies. Her training in pre- and post-natal fitness and physical therapy made me feel at ease. I loved hearing stories from the other women about their own experiences. I continued participating until just over a week before Angelina was born. The exercises made me stronger and helped me learn to trust in my body, which I am sure played a big role in my having an easy delivery. I couldn't wait to get back to the postnatal classes with Angelina. It was a wonderful experience for us both.

I have since recommended the CoreMama™ classes to many other moms-to-be. Now I will recommend *Baby Weight* as well, so they can benefit from Micky's wealth of knowledge and techniques and can learn the CoreMama™ exercises at home!

## MACHTELD AND DIAGO

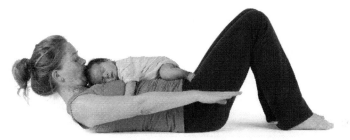

Machteld gave birth to Diago by cesarean only 7 weeks before our first photo shoot. She practiced the CoreMama™ exercises along with strong yoga classes throughout her pregnancy, so her doctor cleared her to start many of the intermediate and advanced level exercises before the more conservative recommendations.

"Having a bad back for years due to two herniated lumbar discs, and having had my first child by cesarean, I knew how weak I could feel during pregnancy and after surgery. Due to this previous medical condition, I was destined for another cesarean. I did a few sessions with Micky to learn exercises to stay strong during my pregnancy. She taught me the CoreMama™ exercises, which I did regularly at home until the last week of my pregnancy. I also continued a strong yoga class weekly until about a month before my baby was born. Under Micky's direction, I started the gentle exercises a week after giving birth, and progressed slowly to include more difficult exercises as my doctor and my body allowed. I felt strong enough to start back to my yoga classes about 10 weeks after having Diago. I was stronger, had less back pain, and was able to lose weight and get back to my normal routine faster the second time around. I would recommend *Baby Weight* to every pregnant woman."

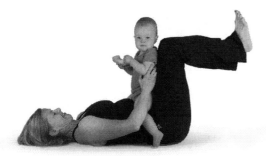

### SHANNON AND ZOE

Shannon discovered the CoreMama™ classes when Zoe was 6 months old. Zoe was just over a year old at the time of the photo shoot.

"What a great concept Micky has developed! The idea to exercise harder than we are traditionally taught throughout pregnancy, then to continue the same exercises with the baby afterward is innovative. Micky's program can help many women who have a hard time finding time to exercise to get an effective workout both during pregnancy and after giving birth by doing the exercises in short spurts. I wish I had discovered it while I was pregnant. Her book is a must-have for expecting and new mothers."

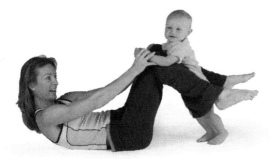

### KATIE AND SANTIAGO

Katie was an original CoreMama™. Santiago had just turned a year old in their photos, but Katie started the CoreMama™ classes when she was about 18 weeks pregnant with him. She delivered Santi via cesarean at 38 weeks.

"I have always had a strong core, but I felt weak for a long while after having my daughter, Tatiana, by cesarean section. Six years later, I hoped for a quicker recovery from my second pregnancy, so I started training with Micky early in the pregnancy. The exercises were gentle but challenging. I trembled in an hour-long class but felt great afterward and was able to maintain and even gain strength throughout my pregnancy. I felt normal again much faster after my second cesarean. I am certain the exercises made a big difference."

## CINDY AND LINDSEY

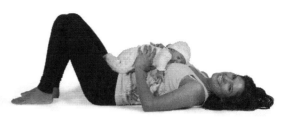

Cindy was 28 weeks pregnant at the time of the first photo shoot. Baby Lindsey was 10 weeks old for the second shoot. Cindy attended the CoreMama™ classes regularly from 16 to 32 weeks. Lindsey was born by cesarean section at 38 weeks.

"The prenatal exercises made a big difference in my second pregnancy. I felt stronger, more fit, healthier and more confident. I found the exercises challenging, and I had to modify them at first, but with time I could do the more difficult variations. It felt great to feel stronger as I grew more pregnant, as compared to my first pregnancy when I felt completely out of shape by the time I had the baby. I found it much easier to lose the weight and get back into exercise and my normal active lifestyle after Lindsey came. I felt confident doing Micky's exercises soon after the cesarean, because she is a medical professional and understood well my condition and needs. I can't wait to share *Baby Weight* with my pregnant friends!"

## MICKY AND MAKANI

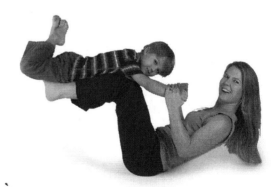

Micky is the *Baby Weight* author. Makani is the original *Baby Weight* baby, the inspiration for the book and the exercises. He was 4 years 10 months old in the photos, and weighed 40 pounds!

"Developing the CoreMama™ exercises, researching and writing the book, teaching the classes, and continuing to do the exercises with Makani long after he was too big to be called a baby, have given me great joy. I have seen the difference *Baby Weight* can make in the lives of many women. It has been a labor of love, much like birthing and raising a child... far more difficult than one imagines, but oh so worth it in the end. I am delighted to share it on a larger scale now. Here you are, world – enjoy!"

# Chapter 1
# Food for Thought

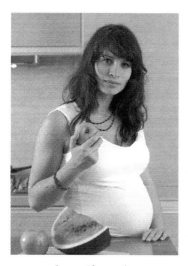

Life is a series of choices. What you choose to put into your body is the most important choice you make during pregnancy and after giving birth. While your body is busy growing a baby, it is essential to follow a healthy and balanced diet to maintain proper nutrient levels not only for growing a healthy baby but also to maintain sufficient energy levels during the taxing, amazing process.

After baby's arrival, the focus shifts a bit but the same principles apply: maintaining nutrient levels for milk production and energy levels for the most demanding job on earth… mothering a newborn. How much weight you gain during pregnancy and how quickly you lose the weight afterward is affected enormously by your food choices.

Pregnancy is certainly not a time to diet in order to try to lose weight. Weight gain during pregnancy is not only normal, it is essential to ensure a healthy baby. You can, however, take control of the pace and, ultimately, the quantity of weight gain by making conscious nutritional choices. A healthy weight gain for a normal pregnancy is 20 to 35 pounds, averaging out at 25 for the mother who was at her ideal weight before pregnancy, on the lower end of the spectrum for the mother who was overweight before pregnancy, and at the higher end for those who were actually underweight before becoming pregnant. In expectant mothers who are markedly obese or underweight, the recommendations vary slightly outside this range.[1] The biology of this weight gain is described in further detail on pg. 43.

There are a few simple principles that can guide you to make informed, healthy choices about what goes into your mouth, and consequently, onto your hips. This is not about deprivation. It is about balance. In balanced proportions, you can eat what you want and maintain a healthy weight gain during pregnancy and have a rapid weight loss afterward.

This is not a diet. This is not a meal plan. This is a way of life.

# First Principle: Eat to Live

It is the simplest but most important of the principles outlined here. View food as your fuel, as the manna from which you derive all your energy and wellbeing. This is, of course, contrary to the philosophy "Live to Eat." When you eat to live, you are conscious of your food choices. This doesn't mean that you don't eat what you want, it means that you also eat what you need.

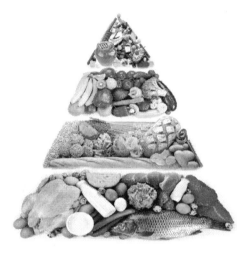

Many expectant mothers fall into the trap of "eating for two." The fact is that your body only needs about 300 extra calories per day to perform the miraculous feat of growing another person in your womb, and that increase is only necessary after the first trimester. Three hundred calories isn't much food, especially if you consume those calories in junk food. You can choose 2 chocolate chip cookies, a small bag of chips, a small order of fries, or a jelly donut, and there are your 300 calories. Some healthier choices still burn up those calories quickly: a plain bagel, a turkey sandwich, and a cup of spaghetti with marinara sauce each weigh in around 300 calories. Of course, those extra calories can amount to a lot more food and nourishment if you make healthy choices: a large mixed green salad topped with a can of tuna or a chicken breast *plus* a cup of fruit salad *and* a square of baker's chocolate for dessert totals less than 300 calories, as does a three egg-white veggie omelet with two slices of whole wheat toast, a half a cantaloupe and a glass of skim milk.

Scatter those extra calories throughout the day as healthy snacks to give you satisfaction and energy all day long. It is the quality of those extra calories, not just the quantity that can make a big difference in how you feel throughout the day, and, ultimately, in how much weight you gain during pregnancy and how fast you lose it afterwards. Eating high-quality, lower-calorie foods in larger quantities makes you feel like you are indulging rather than depriving yourself.

## Suggestions for Eating to Live

Make healthy meal choices in moderate portions and supplement with healthy snacks two or three times a day to stave off hunger. Some suggestions: a handful of almonds or walnuts, carrot and celery sticks, a piece of fruit, a boiled egg, and lean cold cuts rolled around every pregnant lady's favorite, dill pickles!

When you find yourself grazing for a snack or reaching for the fridge, ask yourself what you *need* to eat in that moment. This simple question makes you conscious of your food choice.

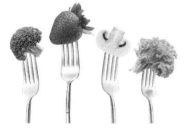

# Second Principle: Eat Fresh

Your mother always told you… eat your vegetables! She was right. Fruits and vegetables provide natural sources for fiber as well as important vitamins and minerals. Oranges and green, leafy vegetables are excellent sources of folic acid, a B-complex vitamin that plays a critical role in the baby's neurological development.[2] Even though you will take a prenatal vitamin supplement, fruits and vegetables should make up 50% of your calories daily. This means that every meal includes a helping of produce and that you are ingesting seven to nine servings per day of the good stuff. Some suggestions to Eat Fresh:

- Eat fruit for breakfast every day
- Drink a can of vegetable juice with an apple for your mid-morning or mid-afternoon snack
- Have carrot sticks, celery and cucumbers in your fridge at all times and serve them on the side with your lunch and dinner
- Eat a big salad nearly every day with 1 of your meals
- Keep steamed or sautéed veggies (squash, onions, peppers, carrots, etc.) in your fridge to add to an omelette or scrambled eggs or serve on the side with any meal
- Make a hearty vegetable soup every week for lunch or dinner from the fridge
- Substitute pasta with steamed mixed vegetables when you eat spaghetti bolognese
- Make a double-sized stir fry of veggies with lean protein at least once a week to have leftovers – get two healthy meals and cook only once

Whenever possible, eat your fruits and vegetables fresh. The nutrient content is much higher in fresh produce compared to canned or frozen and the flavors are much more satisfying, thereby diminishing the urge for sweeter or over-salted processed foods. However, since the availability of fresh produce is largely determined by geographic location and season, remember that the most important part of this principle is to eat the vegetables and fruit, even if they come from the freezer or a tin.

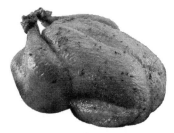

# Third Principle: Eat Lean

This means limit fat intake, and more specifically, be aware of the type of fat you eat. We often unknowingly sabotage otherwise healthy food choices by adding unnecessary fats. Classic examples: a gorgeous fresh salad drenched in a fatty ranch dressing, a lean chicken breast sandwich topped with a thick slice of cheese and a large dollop of mayo, fresh steamed vegetables swimming in butter, pasta primavera with creamy alfredo sauce. I could go on but I think you have the idea.

### Fats: the Good, the Bad, and the Ugly

Fats are essential to a balanced diet, satisfy hunger faster and for longer periods, and provide nutritional benefits not found in other food sources. All fats are not created equal. There is a significant difference between the three main types of fats: saturated, unsaturated, and trans fats.

The unsaturated variety, mono- and polyunsaturated fats, are considered "good" for their numerous health benefits. The American Heart Association suggests that diets richer in these fats actually lower risk for many diseases including heart disease and certain types of cancer.[3] "Good" fats help the body absorb nutrients better, increase nerve conduction velocity, maintain cell membrane health, improve blood cholesterol levels, stabilize heart rhythms, and decrease inflammation.[4] Unsaturated fats are predominantly found in foods from plant sources, such as vegetable oils, nuts and seeds. Some examples of foods rich in monounsaturated fats include avocados, vegetable oils such as canola, peanut and olive oils, nuts such as almonds, pecans and hazelnuts, and seeds including pumpkin and sesame seeds.

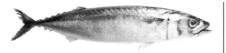

## THE SKINNY ON FATTY FISH

The most common food sources of Omega-3 fats are fish, vegetable oils, and walnuts. Omega-3 fats are particularly of interest to the pregnant or nursing mother as research suggests that from third trimester until age two, a developing child needs a steady supply of DHA, a type of Omega-3 fat found in fish, for healthy brain and nervous system development. This contradicts some recommendations to limit fish consumption during pregnancy due to risk of consuming mercury and other contaminants.

The Harvard School of Public Health points out that evidence for harm to the fetus from a lack of Omega-3 fats is far more consistent than that for the risk of contamination.[5] You can reduce the risk of contamination by consuming a variety of seafood and by avoiding altogether the four types of fish found to be highest in mercury content: shark, swordfish, king mackerel, and tilefish (also known as golden snapper or golden bass). It is recommended that everyone, including pregnant and nursing women, eat two servings of fish per week.[3, 5]

Polyunsaturated fats, including the now well-known Omega-3 fats, are found in high concentration in other oils such as corn, soybean, sunflower, and flax seed oils, and also in walnuts, flax seeds and fish, especially fatty fish such as salmon, tuna, sardines, and shrimp. Dietary consumption of Omega-3 fats is especially important since the body cannot synthesize these fats from other raw materials as it can all other types; they must be consumed in foods or supplements.

Conversely, saturated fats are considered "bad" fats for their undesirable cardiovascular effects, namely lowering the desirable HDL cholesterol levels and raising the artery-clogging LDL levels. Also, the body can synthesize all the saturated fats it needs from other materials, so dietary consumption is unnecessary and should be avoided altogether or at least significantly limited. Saturated fats are found primarily in fatty meats and whole-milk dairy products, but also in coconut and palm oils.

Even worse than saturated fats are trans fats, which come from hydrogenated vegetable oils and are found mainly in processed foods, commercial baked goods, and deep fried fast foods. Trans fats are the "ugly" fats, especially in terms of their effect on the body. Trans fats increase blood levels of LDL cholesterol even more than saturated fats and appear to trigger an inflammatory response in the body, which increases risk of heart disease, stroke, diabetes and other chronic conditions. Evidence suggests that even small amounts of dietary intake of trans fats can increase risk of heart disease by more than twenty percent.[4] Thus the recommendation, avoid trans fats altogether. Your heart will thank you as will your hips. Some suggestions for achieving the "Eat Lean" recommendation:

- Choose lean meats such as chicken breast, pork chops, ground sirloin, and turkey sausages. Trim meat and poultry choices of all excess fat and skin before cooking
- Avoid fatty meats such as marbled steaks, bacon, salami, and sausages
- Eat at least 2 servings per week of low-mercury fish or seafood (see pg. 29 for examples)
- Choose low-fat or fat-free dairy products such as milk, cheese, cottage cheese, cream cheese, and yogurts, and avoid all full-fat dairy intake. Skip the cream and whole milk cheese
- Opt for fresh veggie and tomato sauces vs. the fatty cream sauces
- Avoid fried foods and cut back on fats in cooking. Cook in nonstick pans and use a mister for only a light coat of oil to sauté or fry, or sauté in veggie broth to eliminate the oil altogether
- Eliminate some or all of the yolks from your eggs for breakfast, in tuna salad, or boiled, as snacks
- Replace fat with flavor: Choose full-flavor cheeses to grate and sprinkle lightly over vegetable and pasta dishes. A tablespoon of parmesan adds only two grams of fat but a world of flavor. Cook with plenty of garlic, onion, herbs and spices to make up for the oil and butter you eliminate from fatty recipes
- Make low-fat choices when you can. Use butter substitutes rich in Omega-3 oils on toast and veggies. Choose low-fat or fat-free salad dressings and mayonnaise

Don't be duped by the low-fat packaged food trend. Most of it is sugar-laden and full of empty calories to make up for the lower fat content. The main exceptions are dairy products and salad dressings. Aside from these, stay away. A low-fat chocolate cake will go straight to your hips as fast as the full-fat variety, if not even faster because the fat in regular cake can slow the sugar absorption, a concept further explained in the Fifth Principle: Be Carb Conscious. Highly processed and modified packaged low-fat foods are also far more likely to increase your risk of disease and won't help you lose weight.

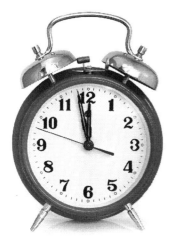

# Fourth Principle: Eat Frequently

Overeating is most often caused by not eating for extended periods of time. If you head off your hunger at the pass, you can avoid this pitfall.

We have all heard that breakfast is the most important meal of the day. Since it is the first meal of the day, it is very important not to skip it entirely. Even if it is only a glass of skim milk and a banana, put something in your stomach within an hour or so of waking to get your metabolism fired up. Have you ever noticed that you seem to feel hungrier after having eaten breakfast than you do if you skip it? That is testament to your body having kicked into a higher gear after the early morning fuel. You probably also notice a clearer mind and more energy.

For most people, it is best to eat a light but satisfying breakfast followed by a mid-morning snack about three hours later. Good breakfast options are fruit and a high-fiber cereal with skim milk, or a veggie omelet made with 1 whole egg and 2 egg whites, and a slice of whole-wheat toast. For snacks, consider:

- High protein, low fat snack bars are a good option for moms on the go, as are nature's perfect snacks, apples and bananas or a handful of nuts
- Lean cold cuts, low fat cheese, and hard-boiled eggs are satisfying snack options
- Drink vegetable juice or skim milk with your snack for a filling burst of nutrients

Have a hearty midday meal with a four to six ounce portion of lean protein and veggies, then have another healthy snack mid-afternoon. By dinnertime you probably won't be too hungry and can eat a light meal without feeling deprived.

During pregnancy, this principle is especially important from the outset since most women find that nausea is avoidable if they eat frequently. The queasiness of the first trimester is sometimes debilitating but can be significantly diminished if not eliminated altogether with a very regular eating regimen. Some women have to eat something every hour to stave off the symptoms. This can also help to combat the first trimester fatigue.

It goes without saying but should be said anyway that if you are going to eat all day long, you *must* make healthy food choices. Otherwise you will gain weight too rapidly during pregnancy and impede weight loss after your baby's birth.

## Fifth Principle: Eat Your Calories, Don't Drink Them

Many weight-loss programs are sabotaged not by what you eat, but by what you drink. Most non-diet beverages, including natural juices, are full of calories.[6] The exceptions: vegetable juice (the low sodium variety is best), black coffee or tea, and, of course, good old-fashioned water.

Drinking a regular soda is like eating sugar out of the bowl. Since a regular cola contains nearly ten teaspoons of sugar, and you want to avoid excessive calorie consumption, you should avoid regular sodas. It is not recommended that expectant or breastfeeding mothers drink beverages sweetened with sugar substitutes since their effect on the developing fetus is unclear.[7] If you have a soda habit that you find hard to kick, try substituting club soda with a splash of natural juice.

You may think you are making a healthy choice having a twelve-ounce glass of

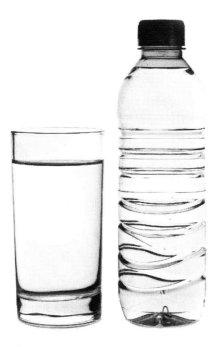

orange juice instead of a soda with your meal. It's true that the juice is natural, not chemical-laden, and contains vitamins that cola does not. And the sugar in the juice is the more favorable fructose rather than sucrose. That juice, however, has the calorie content of sixteen ounces of regular cola. For weight loss or prevention of weight gain, the solution is to skip the juice, replace it with water and have a fresh orange for dessert or your next snack. The whole fruit is always a better choice, because it has fewer calories and higher fiber content. Eating two large oranges provides your body with 30% of the recommended daily intake of fiber and the same 170 calories as a twelve-ounce glass of the juice, which provides almost no fiber. Because whole fruit is filling, most of us couldn't or wouldn't eat two large oranges in a row, while a tall glass of OJ goes down in a flash. The sugar in the juice is absorbed almost instantly into your bloodstream whereas the sugar from the fruit has a time-released effect because the body has to work to break down the fiber before getting to the sugar.[8]

When you are thirsty, drink water. If you have never been a water drinker and it seems far too boring or restrictive to limit yourself to the non-caloric drinks, try sparkling water to make it more interesting, with a couple of ounces of fresh fruit juice to jazz it up if flavor is important.

Alcohol is a big no-no while you are pregnant, and still while you are breastfeeding, mainly for the risk to the baby's health. Even if you are not nursing after your baby's birth, you should drink only in moderation if you want to lose your baby weight quickly. Beer is full of calories *and* sugar, the sugar being maltose, which actually goes into your system even faster than sucrose (table sugar)[8]. Wine is a slightly better option but should be taken occasionally and in moderation when you are trying to lose weight. If you really crave a glass of red wine with your veal parmesan, have one, and stop there.

## Sixth Principle: Be Carb Conscious

Dr. Arthur Agatston described in brilliantly simple terms the physiological process of sugar absorption into the blood stream in his famous book, *The South Beach Diet*.[8] He explains that all carbohydrates contain sugar but that not all carbs are created equal. They differ primarily in how quickly they are broken down and absorbed into the blood. The more rapid-release variety of carbohydrates triggers a subsequent spike in insulin production. The flood of insulin eventually results in a perceived low blood sugar level (hypoglycemia) and increased cravings for more sugar sources, preferably of the sort that gives that quick sugar rush. This inevitably results in overeating and weight gain, which will become a chronic cycle if not addressed.

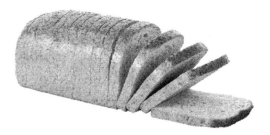

The slow-release carbs, on the other hand, produce gradual rises in blood glucose levels. The insulin levels follow on the gentle curve, rising and falling in balance. What makes a carb release its sugars more slowly? Competition. If a food is pure carbohydrates, i.e. all sugar, it goes straight to the blood on its way to the waist. If the sugars are accompanied by fiber, protein, acidic compounds, or "good" fats, the body has to break down the competing energy sources *on the way* to absorbing the sugar. Some examples of slower-releasing carbs: beans, lentils and other legumes, whole grain pasta, rice, and breads, high-fiber breakfast cereals, and vegetable carbohydrates contained in carrots, tomatoes, squash, and broccoli.

The benefits of fiber intake go far beyond the slowing of absorption of blood sugar. Fiber also has great digestive effects that keep the process moving in a continuous and timely manner and helps the colon to function more efficiently. This is why high-fiber carbs are considered "good" carbs.

As described in detail in the Third Principle: Eat Lean, there are also "good" fats that help reduce carbohydrate effects on the body. The body feels more satisfied by foods that are somewhat fatty. Low fat is a good general diet principle but remember that fat satiates hunger better and for longer, so it can actually do you a favor in preventing weight gain or aiding in weight loss. Consuming moderate amounts of "good" fats with your carbs helps your body process the carbs more effectively. Some suggestions for staying Carb-Conscious:

- Eat only whole grain breads, pastas, cereals, and rice for their high fiber content
- Be conscious of portion size, eating the recommended seven to nine "servings" a day of the healthful whole grain foods described above. Be aware that a "serving" is a single slice of bread or a half-cup of cooked pasta, rice or cereal. You might easily consume four "servings" in a single heaping plate of pasta
- Consume little or no raw sugar, sweets, or sugary drinks
- Balance your carb portions throughout the day. If you have a sandwich at lunch, skip the bread with dinner. If you splurge on a piece of key lime pie, limit all other carb consumption throughout the day to balance out the sugar infusion

# Seventh Principle: Power Up with Protein

Nearly all body tissue, including hair, teeth, muscle, bone, and blood, consists of protein. Proteins are made up of 20 different types of amino acids, 11 of which your body can synthesize, leaving nine that come exclusively from dietary sources. These nine *essential* amino acids are derived from the combination of various proteins that you ingest. During pregnancy, the demands of growing a placenta and a larger uterus, not to mention a *complete person* in the womb, drastically increases the need for proteins. Proteins also play a significant role in various other biological functions, since all enzymes are proteins and are involved in a multitude of biological processes in all of the body's systems. Protein consumption plays an important role in maintaining a gradual, healthy weight gain and loss during and after pregnancy. Protein requires more energy from the body to process, so you actually burn more energy digesting proteins than carbohydrates. Since proteins move more slowly through the digestive tract, specifically from the stomach to the intestines, you feel fuller longer and get hungry later when you consume more protein. Ultimately, like carbohydrates, proteins are converted to glucose to be burned as fuel, but the difference in protein and carbohydrates is that proteins cause a slow and steady release of that glucose into the bloodstream as opposed to the sharp spike associated with carbohydrates, also resulting in fewer hunger pangs afterward.[8]

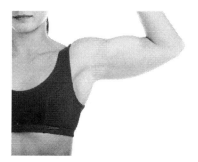

It must be said, in this age of high protein low carbohydrate fad diets, that proteins should not be consumed to the exclusion of all other food groups. Balance is the key to a healthy diet. Fruits and vegetables and whole grains play an important role in fulfilling vitamin, mineral, and fiber needs, and should be consumed in the recommended ranges as well. Quantitative recommendations for protein consumption during pregnancy and lactation vary, with the minimum being around 60 grams per day but with some nutritionists recommending up to 100 grams per day. The most practical recommendation is that expectant and new mothers alike consume three 4 oz. servings per day of lean meat, chicken, or poultry. Non-meat sources of protein include eggs, soy products such as tofu and tempeh, beans and legumes, peanut butter, and dairy products. Be aware, though, that those products must be consumed in greater quantities to equal their carnivorous counterparts in protein power. An egg, a cup of cooked beans, an 8 ounce glass of skim milk, a 4-ounce yogurt, 4 ounces of tofu and 2 tablespoons of peanut butter each provide only 1/3 of a serving of protein, for example.

When choosing your proteins, the most important thing to remember is to look at the whole nutritional package. Some sources high in protein, a marbled steak, for example, are also high in saturated fats. If you plan to get much of your protein from dairy products or peanut butter, their high fat content can be an issue. Some proteins, such as beans, nuts, and whole grains, also provide fiber and other micronutrients that meats lack. And some meats, especially fish, are rich in the "good fats," boosting their overall nutritional power in addition to their high-protein status. Low fat dairy products are also fabulous calcium providers, a big plus for the pregnant or lactating mother. It is best to eat a variety of proteins on a regular basis, to reap the complementary benefits of the various protein sources. In general, animal proteins are more complete in their essential amino acid content. So, if you don't eat much or any meat, it is even more important to eat a wide variety of protein sources. Some suggestions to Power Up with Protein:

- Include a lean protein source in every meal
- Cook extra and store leftovers of fish or chicken to add to a fresh salad to make a quick lunch or dinner
- Drink a glass of skim milk once or twice a day with meals or snacks, or a cup of warm skim milk with a chocolate-flavored vitamin supplement as dessert
- Eat lean cold cuts rolled with low-fat cheese or pickles as filling snacks
- Try cooking meats with low-fat methods (poached, roasted, grilled, etc.)
- Eat hard–boiled eggs for snacks or in salads, and egg-white omelets for breakfast
- Enjoy low-fat yogurt and cottage cheese as snacks or with fruit for dessert

## DAILY INDULGENCE

Any lifestyle based on deprivation will inevitably produce unhappiness. Adopting *Baby Weight's* seven practical and healthy principles will help you to keep your baby weight gain in check and to lose it in short order after giving birth. As with everything in life, it is all about balance. So while you should be continually conscious of your

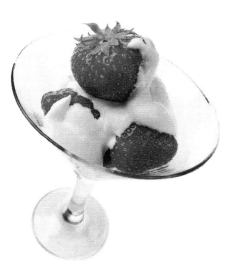

nutritional choices, don't forget to allow yourself to judiciously indulge in that which makes you happy. If chocolate is what makes your taste buds sing, keep a bag of semisweet baking squares or chips in the freezer (they are the lowest-sugar variety). Remove 1 square (or 2 – 3 chips), sit with it and a cup of tea, place it on your tongue and savor the luscious sweetness for as long as it lasts. You will be amazed at how satisfying a chocolate chip can be! Other good choices for daily indulgence are berries or other fruit topped with a dollop of nonfat whipped topping or drizzled with honey, natural sorbets or sherbets, puddings made with skim milk, or a glass of skim milk with a teaspoon of high-vitamin chocolate mix. There are many low fat and low carb dessert recipes out there, but beware of those using artificial sweeteners especially while you are pregnant or breastfeeding. Full-fat and full-sugar sweets should be less frequent indulgences, and always in small sampler portions. If sweets don't really do it for you and it's the savory treats you crave, the same principles apply: if that's what you love, have it but in very small quantities.

A few women in my CoreMama™ classes have complained that they can't do daily indulgence, that the small portions of treats are too difficult and actually leave them frustrated and wanting more. For them, it works better to stick to the seven principles throughout the day all week, then choosing 1 day a week that they can indulge in a full portion of their favorite vice, be it a piece of pie or a plate of fries. To each her own – just remember that the good things in life shouldn't be eliminated completely!

## NUTRITION AND BREASTFEEDING

It is hard to believe, but lactation is actually more taxing nutritionally on the body than growing a baby. A breastfeeding woman needs an additional 500 calories a day for milk production, as opposed to the 300-calorie increase needed during the last two trimesters of pregnancy. If you choose to breastfeed, you have to be aware of your body's needs and not deprive yourself. Otherwise your milk supply will suffer.[9]

Since the composition of breast milk is primarily protein, fat, and water, those elements need to be readily available in the lactating woman for milk production. She will require a 12 – 15 gram per day increase in protein, which amounts to an additional 2 – 3 eggs, 2 cups of milk, 2 ounces of chicken breast, 3 tablespoons of peanut butter, 1 cup of cooked beans or other legumes, 1 ½ cups of yogurt, 1/3 cup of tofu, ½ cup of nuts, or a ½ a cup of cottage cheese.

Most women already come equipped with the fat required for milk production. If pregnancy weight gain is around the healthy average of 25 pounds, approximately seven pounds of that is fat stores available for lactation.[10] So there is no need to increase dietary fat consumption for breastfeeding purposes.

As for fluids, it is recommended that breastfeeding women drink 8 to 10 8-ounce glasses of water per day. A good practice is to have a tall glass of water while you are breastfeeding and to keep a water bottle with you all day long. If you are exercising regularly, you will need more water to make up for fluids lost with activity, an additional 12 ounces per 25 minutes of aerobic activity in not-too hot or humid conditions.

Many healthcare providers recommend avoiding dieting until after a woman stops lactating. While it is true that you should not drastically limit caloric intake during breastfeeding, you can continue to follow *Baby Weight's* seven basic principles, making healthful food choices while lactating to use the extra caloric demand to your advantage and lose your baby weight faster.

## Vitamins and Minerals

A breastfeeding woman loses about 200 to 300 milligrams of calcium per day in breast milk. She needs to replace the loss to avoid the risk of osteoporosis. Calcium requirements while breastfeeding are the same as in pregnancy, 1200 mg/day, which translates to at least three servings of milk, yogurt or cheese daily to meet that need. Most postpartum health care providers recommend that women continue their prenatal vitamins while breastfeeding to ensure sufficient supply of all vitamins and iron.

## Special Considerations for Vegetarians

Vegetarians are at no nutritional disadvantage during pregnancy and lactation as long as they know how to substitute. Increased protein requirements can be met by consuming more milk, eggs, yogurt, cheeses, legumes, and soy proteins like tofu and tempeh, and peanut butter. But remember, these sources must be consumed in higher quantities than their animal-based counterparts due to their lower concentration of proteins. Animal products are an excellent source of vitamin B12 and iron. Vegetarians might need an extra supplement of these nutrients.

Vegan vegetarians, those who don't eat dairy products or eggs, obviously have more limited options in meeting the protein threshold, and must also be more conscious of calcium requirements. Good nondairy calcium sources include soy milk, nuts, legumes, dark green leafy vegetables, and dried fruits.

Every woman should discuss her eating habits with her perinatal healthcare provider, especially if she is following a special or limited diet.

## MEAL AND SNACK PLANNING

You will increase your potential for success at creating and sticking to a healthy diet by planning. If you know in advance the meals you plan to prepare during the week and the foods that you have on hand when hunger strikes, you will be far more likely to make healthy choices.  After all, it's impossible to make the healthy food choice if the only ingredients on hand don't fall into the healthy choices category. Use the wealth of resources available to help you plan. If you don't like the rigidity of a schedule, you don't necessarily have to plan the day by day calendar of what you will cook throughout the week. But you can choose several meal recipes that follow the Seven Practical Principles from your favorite healthy cookbooks, lean cooking websites or magazines and make your grocery list from the recipes. Also use those resources to help you to plan in advance several healthy snacks to have on hand for munching between meals, and add those to your grocery list too.  Try to stick to your list at the supermarket and bypass the rest. You will find that you have just what you need for the week, and you won't have to wonder what to cook or what to snack on when the time comes.

For recipes, tips and ideas on how to incorporate conscious food choices into your everyday routine, tune into BabyWeightTV™ at www.babyweight.tv.

# Chapter 2
# Body Changes During Pregnancy and Childbirth

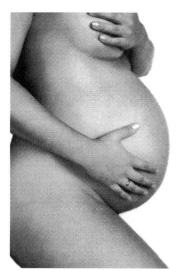

Pregnancy changes everything, including and especially your body. While miraculous and beautiful, pregnancy is also extremely stressful on the body, causing major changes in every system. It is important for the new and expectant mother to understand these changes in order to adapt activities and expectations accordingly.

## SYSTEMIC CHANGES

The circulatory system, for starters, is heavily taxed during pregnancy and therefore undergoes major adaptations. Playing the vital roles of oxygen and nutrient delivery and removal of waste products, this system must accommodate the increased needs of the mother as well as the new demands of the fetus. The body adapts to these demands in many drastic ways. First, overall blood volume is increased by 40 to 45% by the end of a full-term pregnancy, which means the body contains an additional 1.5 liters of blood, creating the stores necessary to accommodate for blood loss during delivery. Plasma volume is increased in greater proportion than iron-containing red blood cells, which carry the oxygen, hence the need for iron supplements during pregnancy to counteract this predisposition to anemia.

The heart, responsible for pumping all that extra blood, responds with increased left ventricular mass and volume and increased stroke volume, the amount of blood the heart pumps with every beat. Heart rate also increases, resulting in increased overall cardiac output. Physiologically, this helps to prevent drastic drops in blood pressure and provides the output needed for increased blood flow to the uterus and fetus. The increased blood volume and cardiac output also enhances the gas and heat exchange between the mother and fetus and enables an increase in circulation to the skin of 4 to 7 times the norm, providing for a more effective cooling mechanism of mother and baby.

Since the pulmonary system is responsible for oxygen intake, this system exhibits similar changes to those seen in the circulatory system in response to the increased oxygen demands of the mother and fetus. Oxygen consumption at rest in pregnant women is increased by up to 32% over non-pregnant women by means of a 40 to 50% increase in the amount of air they breathe. The body accomplishes this primarily by adjusting hormone levels, which control everything, but also with anatomical changes. The ribcage widens and elevates and the diaphragm gradually shifts upward to accommodate more air in the lungs. The diaphragm takes over as the primary breathing muscle. Tidal volume, the amount of air breathed in and out during a normal respiration, is increased, resulting in deeper breathing overall.

## HORMONAL CHANGES

Hormones are the body's chemical messengers. The pregnant and postpartum body is constantly undergoing drastic hormonal changes, which regulate the numerous physiological processes involved in the miraculous feat of growing a baby in 38 weeks. After giving birth, the work continues, all regulated by hormones, to return the body to its prior physical state in roughly the same time frame, while simultaneously producing milk to nourish the new baby.

Estrogen and progesterone levels increase throughout the pregnancy, helping to regulate changes in the breasts and uterus. Levels of Human Chorionic Gonadotropin (hCG) increase immediately in pregnancy, which is why most early pregnancy tests are looking for hCG. hCG is largely related to regulation of progesterone levels. Higher levels of progesterone and relaxin are responsible for the softening of ligaments and other connective tissue throughout the body and have an important effect on the musculoskeletal system.

Hormones control all physical processes, but their effect on mental and emotional states should not be overlooked, and cannot be overstated. The hormonal roller coaster is implicated in the common occurrence of the "baby blues" and in development of more serious postpartum depression. See pg. 60 for more information on this very important topic.

## Body Mass Changes: Your Baby Weight

The pregnant body grows in all directions, but the majority of the expansion is concentrated in the uterus, of course, and the breasts. The uterus expands to more than 10 times its original size and supports a whopping 10 to 12 pounds of weight between the baby, the placenta, and the amniotic fluid. The uterus itself weighs about two pounds more than normal at full term. The breasts increase by up to a pound each. Additional blood volume accounts for three more pounds, and normal water retention another four. Fat stores usually average around seven pounds and are concentrated most heavily around the waist, hips and thighs. All that totals the average 25 – 35 pound weight gain.[10]

## Musculoskeletal Changes

The musculoskeletal system responds to the myriad of hormonal changes, the physical growth of various parts of the body, and the shifting effects of gravity with its own adaptations. From the early weeks of pregnancy, due to increasing levels of progesterone and relaxin, all ligaments in the body become lax, especially those around the pelvis and hips. Ligaments are the connective tissue that stabilizes joints. Therefore, all joints in the body lose some stability. This is especially significant in the sacroiliac joints where the base of the spine meets the pelvis. Many women have dimples over these joints. With instability comes increased movement, which can cause pain. This also applies to the ligaments of the hips, knees, and ankles, where a loss of stability can mean increased susceptibility to damage to the joint structure. It is important to modify activity during pregnancy and during the postpartum phase to account for these changes, eliminating high-impact, jarring movements throughout pregnancy and until around four months postpartum.

## CHANGING EFFECTS OF GRAVITY AND POSTURE

The body's center of gravity is normally right in the center of the pelvis. With the added weight of the expanding uterus growing up and out of the pelvis and into the abdomen, the center of gravity also moves upward and forward. This shift in center of gravity gradually affects balance, causing the later-term pregnant woman to be much less steady on her feet. The abdominal muscles become progressively stretched over the expanding abdomen, weakening their effect as protectors and stabilizers of the lumbar spine. The body relents to these changing forces by developing a more pronounced swayback curve in the lumbar spine, called lordosis. The increased lumbar lordosis, combined with sacroiliac instability, causes the duck-like gait so characteristic of pregnancy. The muscles of the lumbar spine tighten in a compensatory attempt to stabilize the low back, causing a general feeling of achiness and tension in that area.

In response to the increase in size and weight of the breasts, the thoracic spine (mid back) also relents and curves forward, called kyphosis, and the shoulders tend to roll inward while the head moves forward. The muscles between the shoulder blades lose their mechanical advantage and lose strength as they become overstretched. The muscles on the front of the chest and the back and sides of the neck rest in a shortened position and tighten to hold the body further in the altered posture. These anatomical changes can result in tension and pain in the neck and shoulders, in addition to that unsightly hunchback effect. Since these postural changes further weaken the very muscles one would normally use to counteract the effects, thus begins the vicious cycle of weaker muscles causing poorer posture, causing weaker muscles, causing more pain and tension, causing poorer posture, and the cycle continues unless interrupted.

The good news is that nearly all the adverse effects that accompany the physiological changes associated with pregnancy can be prevented, reversed or greatly diminished with regular specific exercise. Stretches and strengthening exercises for thoracic spine extension can reduce the tendency toward kyphosis. Lumbar stretches and abdominal exercises can reduce lumbar lordosis. The CoreMama™ exercises target strengthening the muscles weakened during the normal changes of pregnancy and stretching those that tend to tighten, ultimately minimizing the lasting effects of the body changes.

# Counteracting Postural Changes with Exercise

**Align the cervical spine and reduce neck pain** with neck release stretches and strengthening the neck extensors

**Reverse rounded shoulders** by stretching the chest and shoulder muscles and strengthening the muscles between the shoulder blades

**Reduce low back pain and reverse lumbar lordosis** by strengthening the abdominal corset and back extensors and stretching the lumbar muscles

**Prevent or eliminate Sciatic nerve impingement** with mobilizing stretches for the hips and pelvic girdle

**Improve circulation and prevent leg cramps** with stretches and range of motion exercises for the legs and feet

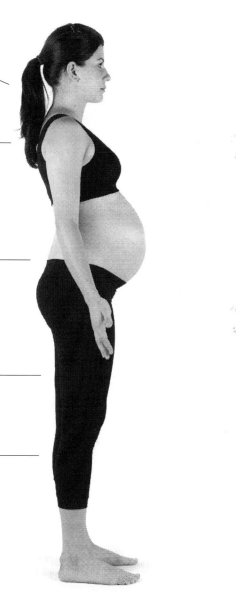

## The Core of the Matter

The majority of the major musculoskeletal changes that occur during pregnancy take place in the body's core, that is to say, in the trunk and proximal muscles and joints, especially the pelvis and hips. The muscular support of the body's core, the core muscle group, is comprised of the abdominal brace on the front and sides, the back musculature from behind, and the pelvic floor down below (see fig. 1,3, and 4).

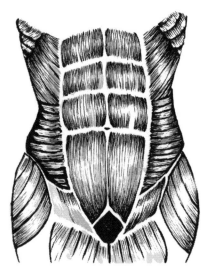

*FIG. 1*

## The Abdominal Brace

Most people don't realize that the abdominal muscles support the pelvis and lumbar spine and that weakness in the abdominal muscles is often the culprit in low back pain. The various layers of abdominal muscles are woven in an intricate meshwork between the ribcage and pelvis to form a corset, which supports the trunk and stabilizes the spine. (see fig.1).

The rectus abdominus muscle is the two-sided superficial muscle whose fibers run vertically, forming that often-sought "six pack" in the trimmest of abs. Its implication in pregnancy is an important one and is discussed later in detail in the discussion of diastasis recti on pg. 47. The internal and external oblique muscles run in opposing diagonal lines, crisscrossing to pull in opposite directions.

Probably the least-known but most important of the abdominal muscles, the transverse abdominus, has horizontal fibers that form a waistband in the space between the lower ribcage and the pelvis. Transverse abdominus muscle tone is a major component in postpartum waistline recovery.

Each of the abdominal brace muscles serves a different function, but it is the combined function of all the muscles that provides stability to the trunk during normal activities and movements. The pull of healthy abs controls the angle of the pelvis in relation to the spine and is responsible for trunk movements in all planes. Activation of the abs braces the body in physically stressful activities, such as lifting or straining, and stabilizes the low back during leg lifts and other activities involving limb movements such as walking. During pregnancy, the increasing weight of the baby in the front places more and more stress on the lumbar spine. The abdominal muscles help to support that weight and protect the low back by maintaining a proper pelvic tilt. After childbirth, abdominal muscle tone stabilizes the spine for the eternal lifting and carrying of the newborn as well as their clingy older siblings, and in recovery of the waistline postpartum.

It is crucial to seek and maintain good abdominal muscle tone during pregnancy to prevent low back pain or injury, to keep erect posture, to have the strength needed to fully engage the abs in the pushing phase of labor, and to bounce back to a firm tummy much faster after childbirth. It is equally important to start specific core-strengthening exercises as soon as possible after childbirth to restore muscle tone, to protect the lumbar spine and reduce aches and pains, and to regain the pre-partum figure. Become a Core-Mama™, fit to the core, with the specific core-focused exercises outlined in chapter 6.

## DIASTASIS RECTI

Diastasis recti is a common condition occurring when the fibrous connective tissue between the two sides of the rectus abdominus muscle splits open. It occurs due to the hormone-induced softening of the tissue itself and the mechanical strain on this weakest link in the abdominal brace. As the uterus grows, the two sides of the rectus abdominus muscle split open like a zipper that gives way under too much strain (see fig. 2).

This separation occurs to some degree in all women. The separation itself is not painful, but a common discomfort in women with more severe cases of dias-

## DIAGNOSING DIASTASIS RECTI

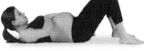

Lying flat on your back with your knees bent, place one hand on your abdomen just above the navel with fingertips pointing downward. Press your low back flat into the floor and slowly raise your head and shoulders. You may see a bulge, but if not you will likely feel the gap between the muscles. If you can only fit 1 or 2 fingers into the gap, there is no reason to modify activity other than avoiding strenuous movements described on pg. 48. If three or more fingers fit into the gap, modify the exercises to avoid increasing the separation and perform specific corrective exercises to help close the gap (see pg. 90)

Due to overstretching and loss of mechanical advantage, the abdominal muscles are virtually paralyzed for 48-72 hours after childbirth. Wait until day 3 after a vaginal birth and day 10 after a cesarean to assess severity of diastasis recti. If you follow the CoreMama™ exercises as part of the *Baby Weight* Fitness Plan, starting day one with gentle isometric exercise, you will be well on your way to closing the gap by day 5. Specific guidelines for exercising with diastasis recti are discussed on pg. 75.

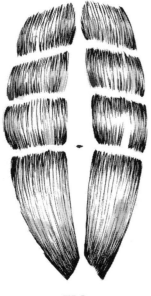

*FIG. 2*

tasis recti is chronic backache in the low back due to loss of strength and stability. The severity of diastasis recti is measured in terms of finger-widths. A separation of less than 3 finger-widths is normal.

It was long believed that women should not do abdominal exercises during pregnancy in order to reduce the risk of diastasis recti. It is now better understood that maintaining good abdominal muscle tone can actually help to reduce the severity of the separation and decrease the recuperation time in closing the gap after birth. However, you must avoid the most strenuous of positions and movements to protect the fragile midline. Lifting or lowering straightened legs is a big no-no, although a modified version (see pg. 108) is perfectly safe. Moving from lying on your back directly up to sitting also puts undue strain on the abdominal wall and should be avoided. Try to always roll to your side first, then push up to sit. Stay within your ability zone with all core exercises and perform only the exercises and only to the degree that you can maintain a strong posterior pelvic tilt (see pg. 88). Following an exercise program devised especially for pregnant and postpartum women by a perinatal healthcare expert is the key to getting and staying strong safely. The Co-reMama™ exercises take all necessary precautions to protect your constantly changing body while providing sufficient challenge to continually make you stronger. See pg. 75 for specific recommendations for exercise with diastasis recti, and tune into BabyWeightTV™ for classes tailored to those needs at www.babyweight.tv.

## The Pelvic Floor

So far we have discussed the effects of supporting the radically enlarged abdomen from the front and the back, but gravity takes its greatest toll on the part down below. The pelvis forms the bony framework for this support (see fig. 3), but the real floor that holds it all up is a meshwork of muscles and connective tissue forming a

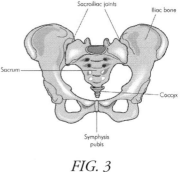

*FIG. 3*

flexible sling, a muscular hammock that holds the vagina, uterus, intestines, and all other abdominal organs in place (see fig. 4).

The muscles form a figure-eight around the three orifices that pierce the midline of the pelvic floor, with top half of the eight encircling the urethra and vagina and the bottom half encircling the anus. Pelvic floor function during pregnancy is especially important as the weight of the rapidly expanding uterus stresses the demand on the pelvic floor. Loss of pelvic floor muscle tone plays a large role in the development of urinary incontinence during pregnancy. For many women, that embarrassing leaking phenomenon persists after giving birth for months or longer. Late in pregnancy, the pelvic floor muscles become overstretched under the load, weakening them further, so they become even more overstretched, making them weaker, and the vicious cycle continues. The cycle can be broken, however, by achieving and maintaining good muscle tone and control of the pelvic floor. Like any other muscle group, you can train the pelvic floor with specific exercises that isolate the muscles.

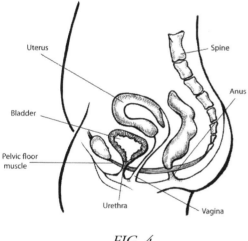

Kegel exercises, named after the doctor who invented them, are an isometric contraction of the pelvic floor muscles. You can practice them by pulling the perineum upward and inward, in the exact movement one uses to stop the flow of urine. That contraction, held for a few seconds at first and progressively prolonging it, builds strength and stability in the pelvic floor. See pg. 51 for specific pelvic floor exercises.

*FIG. 4*

Beyond offering better support for the increased weight of the baby and uterus throughout pregnancy, having good tone and control in the pelvic floor musculature increases elasticity of the vaginal wall, enabling an easier birthing experience and decreasing the risk of perineum skin tears during delivery. A vaginal childbirth puts incredible strain on the pelvic floor muscles, which must relax to allow expansion of the vaginal wall to enable the baby's passage. The muscles become overstretched at best and sometimes even torn during delivery, and oftentimes cut if you underwent an episiotomy. Therefore, some degree of pelvic floor damage is certain after a vaginal delivery. The pelvic floor muscles can be damaged before labor as well, especially if your baby is especially heavy and/or you carrythe baby low for anytime at all, as the constant strain of the baby's weight causes and overstretching of the muscular floor that holds it up. Regular training of the pelvic floor muscles during pregnancy is your best bet at minimizing pelvic floor trauma during pregnancy and childbirth. Consistent training of the pelvic floor postpartum is the key to a rapid recovery down below.

The pelvic floor supports *all* the internal organs from the bottom up. The implications are enormous for all women, especially later in life due to the prevalence of urinary incontinence and vaginal and uterine prolapse in older women. A 2008 study of nearly 2000 women found occurrence of pelvic floor dysfunction in almost 10% of women ages 20 – 39, 26.5% in women 40 – 59, 36.8% of women ages 60 – 79, and 49.7% of women over 80. The study also found similar increases in the incidence of pelvic floor dysfunction with the number of times a woman had given birth, at 12.8% for those without children, 18.4% for those with one, 24.6% for those with two, and 32.4% for those with three or more children.[11] Keeping a strong muscular sling to hold everything in its place is the best medicine to prevent these common conditions.

## PELVIC FLOOR TRAINING – EXERCISES NO ONE SEES

Exercising the pelvic floor is at least as important as any other muscle group, if not even more so. Establishing muscular tone and control in the pelvic floor before it becomes overstretched during childbirth helps prevent urinary incontinence during pregnancy, minimizes trauma to the pelvic floor during childbirth, and helps to speed postpartum recovery.

If the aforementioned aren't reason enough to make a habit of Kegel exercises, there is the added benefit of improved vaginal tone, which can increase sexual pleasure for *both* partners. Legend has it that Dr. Kegel himself, after teaching many women his pelvic floor exercises, was surprised to hear several of his patients report back with markedly increased frequency and intensity of orgasm during intercourse. That good news should make you want to squeeze and hold right now!

The Kegel exercises are, hands down, *the* most important exercises in any prenatal and postpartum regimen, which is why they are incorporated into every stage of the *Baby Weight* Fitness Plan and the CoreMama™ exercises.

## FINDING THE PELVIC FLOOR MUSCLES – THE BASIC KEGEL CONTRACTION

You can identify your pelvic floor muscles easily while urinating by trying to stop the flow of urine. That's it. Squeeze the sphincter of your urethra while you pee, hard enough to interrupt the flow, and hold it for a few seconds before releasing it slowly. If your pelvic floor musculature is already weakened by pregnancy, childbirth, or general lack of use, it may be difficult to achieve a contraction strong enough to actually stop the flow at first. Do your best, holding the strongest contraction you can muster for a count of five, then release. Keep trying. Improvement will be swift. In order to create a functional awareness of the pelvic floor muscles that carries over to activities other than urination, use the urine-stopping exercise only as a learning activity to identify and isolate the pelvic floor muscles, not as an ongoing exercise to be performed every time you urinate, which could irritate the urinary tract and send mixed signals from the bladder to the brain. You can test your ability to stop urine flow about once a week to measure your own progress.

Once you have a feel for it, move on to practicing the Basic Kegel contraction in a variety of positions and situations. The easiest position is lying down, where gravity has little effect. You can progress to sitting, standing, and the most challenging, squatting, as you develop strength and control. After you have successfully isolated the Basic Kegel contraction, begin your pelvic floor training with two types of Basic Kegel exercises:

## EXTERNAL STIMULI, INTERNALLY

In addition to the urine-stopping maneuver, it often helps to have internal stimulation to help isolate the pelvic floor contraction. Since the front half of the figure eight of the pelvic floor encircles the urethra and the vagina, the biofeedback offered by an object placed inside the vagina can be a useful aid in pelvic floor training. You can test your own pelvic floor strength by inserting two clean fingers into the vagina and squeezing the fingers as tight as you can. You can perform the same exercise during sex, squeezing your partner's penis tightly, alternating between Fast Contracts and Slow Holds. While this might become your favorite method of exercising the pelvic floor, don't do it to the exclusion of all others! Diversity is key in developing true control of this muscle group.

There are several types of vaginal weights on the market that offer graduated resistance to the pelvic floor contraction, and make the contraction obligatory in order to hold the weights in place. When you can easily hold a weight in place for an extended time, increase to a heavier weight to increase the resistance and continue increasing strength.

## Fast Contracts

Squeeze and hold the Basic Kegel contraction for just a second before releasing. Hold the contraction just long enough to feel you are squeezing as hard as you can, achieving the maximum contraction. Start with 20 repetitions and work your way up to 100.

## Slow Holds

Squeeze and hold your Basic Kegel contraction for a count of ten, breathing continually. Release the contraction slowly. Repeat for ten reps at first; work up to 50 by adding five reps at a time.

To develop pelvic floor muscle control, practice alternating between fast and slow contractions with ten reps of Fast Contracts followed by ten reps of Slow Holds.

## The Elevator

Once you have gained the strength to do the Slow Hold contraction for ten seconds and ten repetitions, you are ready to move on to this more advanced exercise. To perform the Elevator, start just as you do with a basic Kegel contraction but more slowly and deliberately. In sync with a slow exhalation, visualize an elevator in your pelvic floor rising one floor at a time, with progressively increasing pressure, all the way to the top where you feel you are maximizing the contraction. Hold it at the top through the following inhalation and release it slowly on the next exhalation to lower the Elevator as slowly as it rose, one floor at a time. As you get stronger you can hold the Elevator at the top for another full breath or more. Be sure to maintain calm breathing throughout this exercise. The Elevator can be performed in any position, but is easiest to begin lying down where gravity doesn't take its toll. Later you can do the exercise in sitting, standing, or squatting, and in almost any situation. You will notice later that we incorporate the Elevator into a myriad of other exercises in various positions. Again, the importance of pelvic floor tone cannot be overemphasized.

When you first begin training the pelvic floor, be sure to rest for at least a full minute after the full set of each exercise to avoid overexertion and fatigue of the muscle group. Gradually increase intensity (length of time held and/or effects of gravity) and number of reps as you are able.

# Chapter 3
# Pregnancy and Exercise

The best way to prepare your body for the myriad of physical changes it undergoes during pregnancy and childbirth is to get physically fit before getting pregnant. However, if you were at not at your optimal fitness level when you became pregnant, don't despair. It is never too late to begin. Small changes and efforts now will make big differences from now on.

Staying active during pregnancy helps your body better adapt to and cope with the physical changes and gives you more energy. You can counteract many of the adverse musculoskeletal effects of pregnancy with specific exercises to strengthen what becomes weak and to stretch what becomes tight. You will have fewer aches and pains and feel better overall if you exercise regularly.

## BENEFITS OF EXERCISE DURING PREGNANCY AND BEYOND

Dr. James F. Clapp III has become a pioneer in researching the physiological effects of exercise during pregnancy on the mother and the fetus. His research provides scientific support for what active women have felt all along: that it is perfectly safe and even beneficial for women to become or to stay physically active throughout a normal, healthy pregnancy. His book, *Exercising Through Your Pregnancy,*[12] thoroughly documents the findings of his many years of studies and is an invaluable resource for anyone seeking further knowledge on the subject.

In his studies, Dr. Clapp documented the occurrence of physiological changes in pregnancy which themselves closely resemble the normal physical changes that occur over time with practicing a regular exercise routine, namely increased blood volume, increased cardiac output, increased size of heart chambers, increased blood flow to the skin, and increased oxygen delivery to body tissues. The implication is that pregnancy itself creates a passive training effect that enables the body to meet the new demands of growing a fetus. These effects are compounded by the effects of regular exercise in a way that the fit woman who continues exercise throughout pregnancy can achieve greater benefits from the exercise than if she were not pregnant. This additive training effect appears to last for years after pregnancy in women who stay active after giving birth, indicating that pregnancy might actually give athletes who continue to train throughout pregnancy an advantage, a sharp contrast to traditional views.

The prospects for women who are not already fit but begin an exercise program during pregnancy are also encouraging, in that any training effect achieved through the exercise is combined with the similar physiological effects of pregnancy. According to Dr. Clapp's studies, the results appear to be less pronounced but still significant, and appear to be maximized by regular (five times per week) exercise until the last days of pregnancy.

Aside from the cumulative training effect, or improving overall fitness level, the expectant mother reaps many benefits from regular exercise throughout her pregnancy. Clapp's studies indicate that exercising women gain less weight and deposit less fat during pregnancy, having less baby weight to contend with after baby comes. Those women also have fewer complaints of common discomforts associated with pregnancy and experience fewer medical complications throughout pregnancy. Women who exercise through the full term of pregnancy are no more likely to have premature rupture of membranes or preterm labor than those who don't exercise at all or those who stop exercising earlier in pregnancy. In fact, Clapp's evidence suggests that exercising women have shorter and less complicated labors and require fewer medical interventions during childbirth, and have a faster and easier postpartum recovery than their sedentary counterparts.

## Effects of Prenatal Exercise on Your Baby

Many concerns or reservations about exercise during pregnancy were and still are related to the effect of exercise on the fetus in utero, which was largely unknown until recent years. Thanks to Dr. Clapp's definitive studies of the fetal response to regular maternal exercise, which tracked several indicators including fetal heart rate and behavior during and after exercise, and placental and fetal growth throughout the pregnancy, it is now thought that regular exercise might actually give the baby an advantage in utero. The demands of exercise on the mother's body can actually shunt blood away from the uterus to supply the exercising muscles. But, as previously discussed, the normal physiological changes associated with pregnancy (pg. 41) compensate for the increased demands of the fetus and placenta and appear to be more than sufficient to counteract the shunting of blood to muscles and the increased body temperature levels during exercise.

Dr. Clapp concluded that babies who are routinely exposed to fluctuating blood supply and oxygen levels become accustomed to such fluctuations and are therefore physically more prepared for any greater fluctuations that might occur during the normal stresses or complications of labor and delivery. Indeed, Dr. Clapp found babies born to exercising moms had fewer warning signs or difficulties that would warrant medical intervention during delivery. The studies so far have not revealed a single deficit or disadvantage in babies of exercising mothers. Interestingly, the babies born to mothers who stayed very active several times a week up until the last week of pregnancy were born with healthy birth weights but significantly less body fat, a finding that was still evident in the children's body composition in follow up studies on the same subjects five years later. Could it be that maternal exercise is a factor in reducing the tendency for obesity later in life? We will have to wait for the findings of the long-term studies to examine that correlation further, but it is an exciting implication. Exercising through your pregnancy can benefit you and your baby for years to come.

## SAFETY CONSIDERATIONS AND RECOMMENDATIONS

It is recommended that every woman consult her obstetrician or midwife when beginning an exercise program. Be aware, however, that there is a broad spectrum of perception and opinions about prenatal and postpartum exercise. Traditional conservative attitudes have been challenged in recent years and are definitely changing, but more slowly in some areas than others. The expectant mother's desire to become or to stay active may be met with resistance or reservation from more conservative healthcare providers. If you feel the attitude is not in line with your wishes and with modern perception, feel free to voice your concerns and desires to your practitioner and do so with scientific support.

The American College of Obstetrics and Gynecology (ACOG) recommendations for prenatal and postpartum exercise have been revised in recent years to allow for more liberal interpretation.[13] The following *Baby Weight* recommendations are in line with the ACOG guidelines and are supported by Dr. Clapp's extensive research on real mothers and infants.

# Recommendations for Exercise During a Healthy Pregnancy

**Listen to your body.** Keep all activity at a moderate intensity and don't push any exercise to the point of pain or overexertion. A good gauge for cardiovascular intensity is the talk test: if you can still carry on a conversation while exercising, you are in the safe zone. If you are too breathless to talk, take it down a notch. Stretches should be kept in the "pleasantly pulling" part of the spectrum. Strengthening exercises should feel challenging but do-able. Be careful not to overheat; hydrate often and take frequent rest breaks, especially when exercising in hot or humid climates. If you experience any symptoms like dizziness, breathlessness, or profuse sweating, stop exercising and seek shade or a cool environment and take a rest.

**Make a habit of exercise.** It is safer and more effective to engage in a regular exercise routine than to have a more sporadic schedule, because your body is accustomed to the activity and the training effects are cumulative if exercise is done on a regular basis. We recommend that the pre- and postpartum mother engage in some sort of exercise four to five times a week, preferably combining at least 20 mintues of cardiovascular activity with 15 to 20 minutes of CoreMama™ exercises.

**Avoid prolonged periods of back-lying.** Because the baby's weight can compress the major blood vessels which return blood to the heart and provide blood supply to all internal organs, including the uterus, it is recommended that women more than 4 months pregnant not lie completely supine (flat on the back) for more than a few minutes at a time. It is perfectly safe to do exercises on your back, however, if you are changing positions frequently. Also, changing the angle of the pelvis by as little as 15 degrees relieves the pressure on the artery, so just place a pillow under one buttock to shift your baby's weight to one side if you want to practice one of the back-lying positions for more than 2 minutes.

**Choose appropriate activities.** Cardiovascular activities and all other exercises should be fun and safe. If you were already active before pregnancy, it is generally safe to continue your previous activities. Some activities are not recommended for any pregnant woman, however: those that have risk of falling or abdominal trauma such as downhill skiing, horseback riding, and contact sports including soccer, hockey, and basketball. Women who were already running regularly can continue to do so well into pregnancy, but those who were not should stick to walking or to an elliptical machine since the body is not used to the repetitive impact. Anyone who is not on bed rest can safely walk or swim, regardless of prior activity level, which makes these two the author's favorite cardio activities during pregnancy.

**Include a warm-up and cool-down in every exercise session**. Starting slowly allows the body's tissues to warm up, reducing the risk of injury or post-exercise aches and pains, and also helps the heart rate to rise slowly and safely. A cool-down period ensures a gradual decrease in the heart rate and allows the tissues to settle after the activity before coming to a full stop. See pg. 78 in the exercise section for recommendations on specific warm up and cool down activity recommendations.

**Increase fluid and caloric intake**. To account for the increased caloric and fluid demands of exercise, be sure to always give your body what it needs. In addition to the 300 calories a day your body needs during the second and third trimesters of pregnancy to grow a baby, if you are exercising you also need to replace the additional calories burned with exercise, which will vary depending on the activity but will likely reach 200 calories or more if you are doing the recommended 20 – 30 minutes of cardio training. You will need to drink an additional half a liter of water for every 20 minutes of cardiovascular exercise. Drink before, during, and after exercise to avoid dehydration. In hot or humid weather you will need even more fluid to stay hydrated.

**Exercise in an appropriate environment.** Choose wisely *where* to do your daily workout routine. Surfaces for sitting and lying exercises should be padded with a rug and/or an exercise or yoga mat. If you live in a hot or humid place, outdoor activities should be performed in the cooler hours of the day and in the shade as much as possible. Be sure to wear clothing that suits your particular activity and climate.

# Contraindications to Exercise

There are certain conditions or symptoms that make it unsafe to exercise during pregnancy. The following conditions are considered "absolute contraindications to aerobic exercise during pregnancy" according to the ACOG opinion number 267 published in 2002 and reaffirmed in 2009:[13]

- Preterm Labor
- Ruptured Membranes
- Persistent Bleeding in 2nd or 3rd Trimester
- Placenta Previa after 26 weeks gestation
- Incompetent Cervix/ Cerclage
- Preeclampsia/ Pregnancy Induced Hypertension
- Hemodynamically Significant Heart Disease
- High Risk Multiple Gestation Pregnancy
- Restrictive Lung Disease

The ACOG also listed conditions that warrant termination of exercise while pregnant:

- Preterm Labor
- Vaginal Bleeding
- Amniotic Fluid Leakage
- Decreased Fetal Movement
- Pain or Swelling in the Calf Muscles (to rule out Thrombophlebitis/ blood clots)
- Shortness of Breath Prior to Exertion
- Dizziness
- Headache
- Chest Pain
- Muscle Weakness

Anyone experiencing any of the aforementioned symptoms should stop all exercise and contact a health professional immediately to rule out more serious complications. Your health practitioner can advise you as to which type of exercise are safe.

# Chapter 4
# After Baby Comes – Postpartum Reality

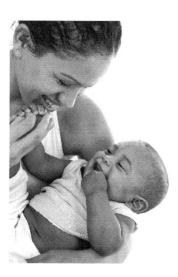

It must be a byproduct of the hormonal imbalance, but most pregnant women harbor the irrational notion that a few weeks after giving birth they will be back in their favorite jeans and overjoyed in their role as new mother. Then they have the baby. No matter how you do it, childbirth is never fun and never easy and always leaves your body over-stretched, over-stressed and over-tired. If you were fortunate enough to have a vaginal delivery, you are likely feeling out of form inside and out. And if you had a Cesarean, you are recovering from major surgery *on top of* recovering from the cumulative effects of nine months of pregnancy.

The postpartum physique is profoundly affected by the awesome feat of pregnancy and childbirth. Face it, your body has been through the wringer. Abdominal muscles that were stretched over the uterus are practically paralyzed for the first few days after giving birth and recuperate slowly thereafter because they lose their mechanical advantage once they are no longer pulled taut over the womb. The perineum and pelvic floor muscles are severely over-stretched and perhaps even torn or cut if you underwent an episiotomy. The postural changes that crept up on you during pregnancy persist, especially the forward head, rounded shoulders hunchback effect and the exaggerated lumbar swayback curve. Ligaments and connective tissue are still lax due to continuing hormonal changes. You are likely to have an achy low back and a very tense neck and shoulders.

Your new job mothering a newborn infant requires a lot from your battered body. The lifting, changing, bathing, pacing, rocking, bouncing, twisting, carrying, and nursing takes its toll on the already weakened and sore body. There is no time to rest and recover. The acute aftermath pains of having given birth are soon replaced by all-over aches and discomfort.

It is not all grim, though – there is some good news! Implement the CoreMama™

exercises (pg. 77) to counteract adverse body changes and get your body back. With diligence, you will see and feel results fast! See Chapter 7: Soothing Mommy's Woes on pg.173 for specific exercises for common prenatal and postpartum aches.

## GENERAL GUIDELINES FOR POSTNATAL EXERCISE

The recommendations for prenatal exercise outlined on pg. 56 also apply to the postpartum period, with the exception of the limitation on time spent lying on the back. There is no such limitation for the new mother. The following list is a quick review of those recommendations:

• Listen to your body and exercise within your limits. Start activity slowly. If you experience an increase in bleeding in the early postpartum days after exercising, you might need to back off the exercise for a few days. That is your body's way of telling you to slow down.
• Always start with a warm up and finish with a cool down activity (see pg. 78 for suggested activities).
• Choose activities appropriate to your fitness level and your environment, dressing appropriately for the activity and the climate.
• Exercise on a regular basis, at least four to five times per week. Include 20-30 minutes of cardiovascular exercise at least three times a week.

## POSTPARTUM DEPRESSION AND EXERCISE

The first days after baby comes are a whirlwind of mixed emotions. Elation, fear, exhaustion, relief. There are many factors at play. The new mother is often abruptly stricken with a harsh new reality that only remotely resembles the romantic images she had when anticipating the arrival of a new baby. She may have difficulty identifying her expectations as unrealistic and accepting the reality of her situation once living it. Then she is faced with meeting the countless demands of a newborn and adjusting to the rigorous round-the-clock schedule, and the inevitable sleep deprivation.
Many women have negative feelings about their body image after giving birth. Feeling isolated and homebound and that they never have a moment to themselves leads many new mothers to feelings of desperation and depression. The dramatic fluctuations in

hormones that occur during pregnancy and after childbirth can further enhance feelings of anxiety and despair.

Women are not generally encouraged to talk much about the negative aspects of new motherhood. They often repress their negative emotions and grin through gritted teeth, feeling the social pressure to rejoice in the experience of expecting or having a new baby. In recent years, doctors and the media have given more attention to postpartum depression as a widespread issue that affects women of all social classes and walks of life, creating more public awareness of the condition.

Postpartum depression encompasses a wide range of symptoms and experiences, from the common "baby blues" to more serious cases of clinical depression, or worse still, postpartum psychosis. Common symptoms are tearfulness, anxiety, nervousness, recurring thoughts and fears about the baby's wellbeing, and lack of interest in outside activities. It is considered normal for women to feel overwhelmed and even quite desperate in those first weeks after giving birth. Up to 80% of women experience the "baby blues" within the first few days postpartum. For that reason, it is often difficult to identify when the feelings cross the line to more serious cases of depression. The "normal" postpartum blues usually subside untreated within two to three weeks. If symptoms persist beyond that time frame, or if the initial symptoms are severe and especially worrisome, you should tell your doctor or midwife and seek help. As many as 12% of new mothers develop postpartum depression, a serious medical condition with significant implications for mother and baby that should be treated as early as possible to minimize the negative impact. Treatment options may include medication to counteract the chemical causes and psychotherapy or counseling to address contributing life issues.[14, 15] Recent studies suggest that 10 to 18% of pregnant women exhibit depressive symptoms,[16] suggesting that postpartum depression might also be an unrecognized prenatal problem.

Exercise is a natural aid in battling the baby blues or even more serious cases of depression, for a variety of reasons. Chemically, the performance of regular exercises lowers blood levels of cortisol, the stress and depression hormone. Exercise also causes an endorphin release; increasing levels of this feel-good hormone gives you a natural high. Also, just the simple act of *doing something* to counteract the body changes associated with pregnancy can go a long way toward boosting self-image. Much research has been done in recent years to investigate the effects of exercise on postpartum depression. Factors and conclusions vary, but nearly all research indicates benefits of exercise on maternal wellbeing to some degree. A 2004 Australian study found that women who participated in a 12-week stroller walking program with other mothers exhibited statistically significant decreases in depressive symptoms and increases in fitness levels compared to the control group that attended a mother's social support group for the same time frame.[17] An extensive study published in 2010 involving 161 mothers over seven years, found that the proportion of women at risk for postpartum depression was decreased by a whopping 50% after eight weeks participation in a mother-and-baby exercise program as compared with the control group.[18] Now there is a yet another reason to pick up your baby and get moving! Find a CoreMama™ or other class near you! Visit BabyWeightTV™ to find the class that suits you best at www.babyweight.tv.

# Chapter 5
# And Baby Makes Two: Including Your Baby in Your Postpartum Recovery

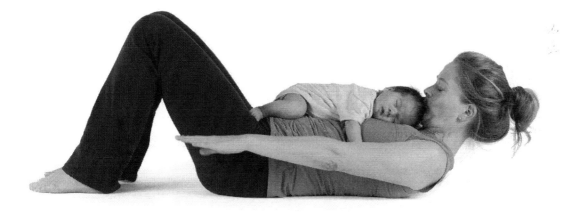

## YOUR BABY'S DEVELOPMENT

Though taxing, the first days, weeks, and months mothering a newborn are marked by a new sense of wonder and discovery through the eyes of a new life. You will likely be mesmerized by the growth and development of your amazing new addition. In the beginning, your baby is completely dependent on you for its every need. After 9 months in your womb with sound of your heart beating her sole source of soothing, your newborn will be happiest held close to you, where she can feel, hear, and smell you.

Babies are born with little to no controlled movement due to weakness and lack of muscular coordination. During the first few months, babies become more aware of and more in control of their bodies. The development of new skills is marked by the achievement of certain motor milestones. The first year's major motor milestones are outlined below, especially focusing on those that relate to the postnatal exercises that follow. Since the *Baby Weight* Fitness Plan is for mommy and baby, I have included handling techniques and activities that I have developed in my work as a neonatal and pediatric physical therapist to help babies progress in motor skill development. Remember that all babies are different and it is normal to have a significant variation from the average in the development of some skills. Premature babies will often achieve most, if not all, first year motor milestones behind their full-term counterparts. Voice any concern over your baby's progress to your pediatrician for further evaluation.

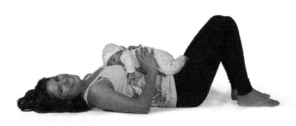

## Developmental Milestones
### 0 – 4 Months
*Sight*
Babies are born with the physical ability to see the world around them, but their brains aren't yet capable of processing complex visual information. They develop this ability gradually over the first 8 months of life. In the first week, newborns can only see about a foot away, making your face the most interesting thing in sight. In the weeks that follow, the ability to focus on further-away objects develops. Around two months, your baby can focus on and track objects, as well as distinguish colors and more complicated patterns. By 4 months, your baby can see well enough to recognize objects that interest her, and has sufficient hand-eye coordination to be able to reach for and grasp for those objects.

**What You Can Do:** Hold your baby close for face-to-face time in the first weeks. Place high-contrast patterns, like checker boards or zebra stripes, close to her in her crib or seat in the first two months. From two to four months, offer her colorful books and toys and encourage her to track the objects that interest her by moving them slowly in front of her. Place her under a baby gym during the same time frame to integrate hand-eye coordination as she begins to bat at objects. This is a great activity for encouraging your baby's development while you do some of the postnatal CoreMama™ exercises that don't involve the baby. Play with rattles and other toys to peak her interest, then place the toys in your baby's hands to encourage her to grasp and to further develop hand-eye coordination.

### *Head and trunk control*

The neck muscles slowly gain strength to help your baby support and control the weight of her head. By three months, she can probably lift and hold her head up while on her tummy and control her head for short periods, albeit in a wobbly fashion, while supported in an upright position. By four months, she can likely hold her head in line with the body when pulled up to a sitting position and hold her head steady when upright for longer periods. She can probably also push up onto her arms while on her tummy, and she may even start to roll over, usually first from tummy to back, at around four months (though this often happens later).

**What You Can Do:** In the first few weeks, it is important that the baby's head is well supported at all times to avoid strain or other injury. It is never too early for tummy time, though, so be sure to give your baby plenty of the prone position to help develop the neck extensors. Consult your pediatrician about on-the-tummy as a sleeping position, usually not recommended until after she can roll over. After the first few weeks, you can help your baby develop head control by propping her in a semi-seated position, resting against your torso as she faces forward or up on pillows with plenty of padding around her. At about three months you can begin to pull her up slowly by her arms from lying on her back, encouraging her to fight gravity to hold her head up in line with her body. Never leave your baby unattended in case she becomes one of the early rollers.

**What You Can Do:** Once your baby has good head control, support her in the seated position on your lap, holding her with both hands on the pelvis so that your thumbs come together on her lower back and the fingers on the forward crests of her pelvis. You have control of her base but she must use her trunk muscles to hold herself upright. Position your baby in sitting on the floor with pillows all around for safety, showing her how to support her weight on her hands in front of her. As she masters this position, place tempting toys in reach that will make her want to lift a hand and shift her weight, further challenging her balance and trunk control.

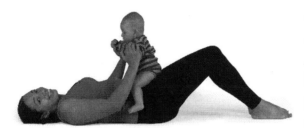

**4 – 8 months**
*Sitting*
After head control is perfected and your baby can roll in both directions, usually from four to six months, she develops the trunk control to be able to hold herself upright when seated. Most babies begin to sit momentarily without support from 5 to 6 months and can move themselves to a seated position and sit steadily without support for longer periods of time around 7 months. By 8 months, the skill is usually perfected and becomes just a transition pose for moving into all-fours or standing in preparation for mobility.

*Crawling*
Once able to sit comfortably and shift the weight forward onto the hands, it is not long before most babies discover how to start to move themselves. Many learn to scoot on their bottoms and use that as the preferred means of locomotion for a time. Others figure out how to pull themselves around on their bellies and remain "combat crawlers" for a while. Eventually, when they develop enough trunk control and hip stability, most babies figure out how to get into the quadruped (all-fours) position and learn to crawl. The time frame for crawling varies widely, but by 8 months most babies are moving themselves rather efficiently in at least one of the three aforementioned ways. It may be as late as 10 or 11 months before your baby crawls, or she might be one of the few that goes straight from scooting to walking.

**What You Can Do:** After she has good sitting balance, while your baby sits with hands supporting her in front, help her to shift her weight forward onto the hands, gradually lifting the weight off her seat. From prone position, place your hands under your baby's hips and pull the pelvis up and back to move her into a hands and knees position. Also from the prone position, bend one knee up and out to the side then lift her pelvis to shift her weight toward that knee to encourage her to take weight into the knee. Later, position her on all-fours while supporting her belly with one hand, then slowly start to reduce the support under the belly, forcing her to hold her tummy up off the ground. Once she is steady on hands and knees, entice her to move forward by placing her favorite toys just out of reach.

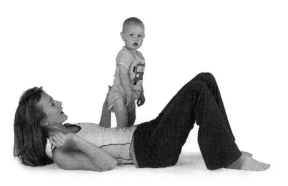

### 8 – 12 months
### *Standing*

By 8 – 9 months, most babies can pull themselves up to stand, can stand while holding onto a surface, and may even be able to make side-steps while holding on ("cruising"). By 11 months, many babies are expert cruisers and can stand unsupported for a few seconds at a time.

**What You Can Do:** First, support your baby from the pelvis while she stands with her hands on a stable surface (a coffee table is usually the perfect height), then shift her weight from side to side to stimulate muscle contraction and prepare for movement. Later, progress to let your baby hold your fingers to support her in standing, again shifting her weight from side to side. She will most likely want to make steps.

### *Walking*

Once they are able to cruise efficiently, it is only a matter of time before babies will get the courage to let go of a surface to try to traverse a distance before arriving to the next support. Many babies accomplish this feat before completing their first year, though most require a couple of more months to become real walkers.

**What You Can Do:** Walk with baby holding your fingers, careful to bend your knees sufficiently to protect your low back, and gradually decrease the support you provide with your hands. Push toys that offer support are great during this phase, too. I personally do not recommend walkers because they don't help babies develop the proximal muscle control they need to balance and walk, and they give them mobility that they are not yet ready for cognitively. I have seen many injuries resulting from walker use.

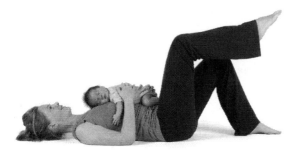

## Incorporating Baby into Your Exercise Routine

**0 – 4 months:** At this early stage, before your baby can move herself, it is easy to integrate her into a series of postnatal exercises. She is probably most comfortable in your arms or somehow in contact with you. You can position your small infant across your chest or tummy, or propped on your legs when lying with your knees bent, to perform a variety of abdominal exercises. With appropriate head support, you can use your baby's weight as resistance during sitting, standing and lying-down exercises. Position her lying on her back or her tummy in front of you while you are lying on your side, or underneath you while you are on all fours or in a lunge position, so that you can interact with her while exercising, taking advantage of the fact that she can't yet mobilize to get away. For some cardio work, place your baby in a front-carrier with adequate head support or in a reclined stroller and take off for a brisk walk. The fresh air will do you both some good. Avoid running with your baby in a jogging stroller until your baby is at least 4 months old and has good head control.

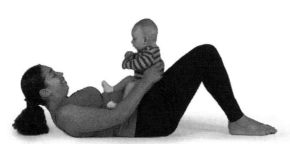

**4 – 8 months:** During this phase, your baby is far more alert and aware of her surroundings. By now she has good head control and is developing good trunk control. She will begin to move herself during this phase, especially through rolling and scooting and perhaps even crawling. Things get more interesting when baby gets mobile. Once she is able to sit supported, you can position her on your pelvis or abdomen, either straddling you or sitting side-saddle, using your hands to support her. She might stay there happily for a few abdominal exercises. You can continue to use your baby's weight for resistance with many exercises, which you will find increasingly more challenging, the heavier she gets. At this age, she will likely enjoy the interaction during exercise even more than before.

When your baby begins to sit unsupported, you can position her in sitting alongside your yoga mat, with plenty of padding all around to ensure a soft landing if (when) she falls, helping her to get her own exercise while you do yours, as she develops the trunk control necessary to become a stable sitter. If she becomes an early crawler, you might have a hard time keeping your baby in the close vicinity while you exercise. In that case, try to engage her for as long as possible in a variety of positions and exercises, then let her free to roam. If you are in an enclosed and childproof area, you can continue your routine while she explores. She will most likely come back to join you shortly.

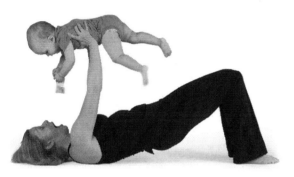

**8 – 12 months:** By this stage all babies become very mobile in one form or another, be it scooting, crawling, or walking. They will still delight in interacting with mom for many of the exercises, but often only on their own terms. At this point, it is best to respect your baby's free will and let her do her thing while you do yours. If you go about your business, she will most likely come around off and on to see what you are up to and to participate for a short time before pattering off again. Surround yourself with her favorite toys, or better yet, take out toys that she hasn't seen for a day or two, to try to keep her near. If she likes a particular video, try playing it while you work out with her.

Your baby can still participate in the CoreMama™ exercises as she is willing, especially seated on your pelvis or on your feet for some lying-down exercises. Strength-permitting, you can continue to use your baby's weight for resistance during all the exercises. If you have been practicing this all along, she won't feel so heavy now!

## INCORPORATING YOUR EXERCISES INTO BABY'S ROUTINE

You may have it all planned, to exercise from 9 to 10 a.m., between feedings and before you have to take the dog to the vet. All appears to be going well, on schedule, when for no apparent reason, your baby rebels. She will not cooperate, let alone participate, in your plan. Depending on how far you are into the motherhood experience and whether it is your first ride on this train, it might be hard to accept that sometimes that's just how it is, that sometimes it doesn't matter what you plan or what big ideas you might have, your baby may have her own agenda. Ultimately, it is she who will control the dynamic of the exercise sessions if you want her to be a part of them.

Be prepared with distractions: toys, books, colorful fabrics, mobiles. If your baby likes a particular video or music, put it on as that might help too. If you can buy yourself even just a few minutes, you can get a lot accomplished. Try changing positions if she gets fussy, moving from sitting to standing to lying on your back to lying on your side. Switch to those exercises that you know are her favorites if she gets bored or restless, even if it means repeating the same exercises. You may only get in a few minutes here and there with your baby and then have to do the other exercises without her while she naps or plays happily doing her own thing. If she flat-out refuses, don't push it. You don't want to sour the experience for her forever. Just gently bring her back to it when she is ready. It is a good idea to have a medicine ball or other 8 – 10 pound weight to use for resistance when baby is not willing to participate, if you are already used to the added challenge of using your baby's weight.

You will find helpful tutorial videos on BabyWeightTV™ for tips on how to incorporate your baby into your exercises, at www.babyweight.tv.

# Chapter 6
# Get Moving!

Now that you understand the physiological changes that take place during and after pregnancy and the risks and benefits associated with prenatal and postpartum exercise, you are ready to get moving! There is no better prescription than the *Baby Weight* Fitness Plan for getting fit during and after pregnancy. It's quite simple really: a healthy diet combined with regular cardiovascular activity and specific core-focused exercises at least 4 days per week. If you follow this plan, you will feel stronger, have more energy and will see results in less than a month.

## The Baby Weight Fitness Plan

**Follow a Healthy Diet:** Adopt the 7 principles in Chapter 1: Food for Thought, to help keep your baby weight gain in the healthy range of 20 – 35 pounds and to speed the weight loss after giving birth. You will also have the added benefits of having more energy and feeling better overall when you make conscious food choices.

**Get in the Zone:** Do some sort of cardiovascular activity for 20 – 40 minutes 3 – 5 times a week. Choose an aerobic activity that elevates your heart rate to the target heart rate zone and keeps it there throughout the activity. The American Heart Asscociation recommends that you aim to increase your heart rate to between 50 and 85% of your maximum heart rate, which is calculated by subtracting your age from 220. If you are pregnant or in the first 2 months postpartum and starting aerobic exercise for the first time in a long time, be sure to consult your healthcare provider first and begin slowly with only 10 – 15 minutes in the 50 – 70% of maximum heart rate zone.

Walking, swimming, biking, dancing, jogging, gym equipment such as the treadmill, rowing, and elliptical machines all provide good options. Other examples of low-impact cardio activities: hiking, low impact aerobics classes, and walking the stairs. Running, jogging, and other high-impact activities are only recommended if you have been practicing that same type of exercise continually throughout your pregnancy. Otherwise, it is best to wait until 4 months postpartum when the hormone levels normalize to begin higher-impact cardio exercise to avoid risk of injury due to joint instability.

Most importantly, do what makes you happy. Choose activities that you like and can easily fit into your daily routine. A brisk walk around your neighborhood or the mall can be as beneficial as a trip to the gym to use the treadmill or the elliptical machine. Don't put off cardio activity until you have a whole hour to devote to going to the gym. Even 8 or 10 minutes of activity a few times a day will help get you in shape. When you have a moment, do a few fast laps around the lobby of your office building or the parking lot, or go quickly up and down a flight of stairs 10 times. It all counts. In fact, varying your activities can make you fit faster because using different muscle groups challenges your body in new ways. For maximum results, step up the intensity of your cardio workout regularly by increasing the pace of or adding arm movements to any activity, adding resistance on the bike or elliptical machine, inclining the treadmill, choosing an interval training program with speed burst segments on a variety of cardio gym equipment, or adding your baby's weight by walking with her in a front carrier or pushing her in a stroller.

**Get to the Core of the Matter:** Train your core muscle groups 4 – 5 days a week. Most of the body changes that occur with pregnancy and childbirth are in the core muscles. The CoreMama™ exercises (pg. 77) specifically target the key muscle groups that weaken during pregnancy. Start training before or during pregnancy to minimize the postural changes and weakness. After baby comes, you can include her in the fun as well by exercising your core with your baby! Start with the beginner level exercises and progress up to the intermediate and advanced levels as you are able. Even just 10 minutes a day goes a long way toward preparing the pregnant body for childbirth and a speedy postpartum recovery. Work up to a 25 – 30 minute session 4 or 5 times per week to become a CoreMama™ yourself.

**Don't Forget your Pelvic Floor:** Integrate Kegel Exercises into every aspect of your life. Do them at stop lights, while waiting in line, while walking, while driving, while talking on the phone, and while doing the CoreMama™ exercises. You cannot overdo them! Alternate between the Elevator, Fast Contracts, and the Slow Hold (see pg. 51). Do at least 100 a day to achieve and maintain pelvic floor muscle tone.

**Relax, already:** Be sure to include relaxation techniques in the warm up and cool down period every exercise session, or at some point during the day, every day. Take just 3 to 5 minutes to focus on your breath and connect with yourself by disconnecting from the mind. The benefits to your own health and wellbeing, as well as to that of your baby, are enormous. See pg. 79 for suggestions on how to relax already.

## WHEN TO BEGIN

Review the guidelines and contraindications to prenatal and postpartum exercises listed on pg. 56-58 and pg. 60, respectively. Talk to your doctor or midwife before beginning any new exercise program to be sure that you don't unknowingly have any conditions that might be considered contraindications to some types of exercise.

After an uncomplicated vaginal birth, you can begin with Kegel contractions and the isometric abdominal exercises (Pelvic Tilt, Activation of Transverse Abdominus) the first day postpartum. On the third day, you can assess for Diastasis Recti. If you have a gap of 3 finger widths or more, you can begin the corrective Splinting exercise and progress following the guidelines listed on pg. 75. If the gap is less than three finger widths, you can start the Beginner exercises in each position on day 3 postpartum.

You can begin the *Baby Weight* Fitness Plan at any point during your pregnancy or after baby comes, as long as you don't have any contraindications to exercise and exercise at the appropriate level. The CoreMama™ exercises are arranged by position: Supine (on your back), SideLying (on your side), Quadruped (on all fours), Sitting, and Standing. Within each position there are Beginner, Intermediate and Advanced exercises. When you begin the program, start with the Beginner Level in each position, progressing to add the Intermediate and Advanced exercises as indicated in the "Progression" section of the description of each exercise. Unless otherwise indicated, start with 10 reps of each exercises and work your way up to 20. Move from one level to another in a particular position after you are able to do the full 20 reps (or otherwise indicated) of all exercises in the level in that position. Unless indicated, don't stop the Beginner Level exercises when you progress to higher levels. Instead, decrease the reps to 10 and use them as a warm up for the more difficult exercises. Kegel contractions are integrated into most of the CoreMama™ exercises. See pg. 52 for a review of the different types of Kegel exercises.

## After a Cesarean

If you had a Cesarean, first and foremost follow your physician's specific advice of when to begin an exercise program. *Baby Weight* recommends not attempting any exercise until 10 days post-op to give your incision time to mend in its most fragile time. You might find relief in wearing an elastic abdominal support during that time frame. Most doctors require a follow up visit around 8 – 10 days post-op and again at 6 weeks post-op. Ask your doctor at those check-ups what you are allowed to do in the weeks that follow. Take *Baby Weight* to show the doctor or midwife the specific exercises with the variations indicated for women who had a Cesarean. When you are approved to begin the CoreMama™ program, follow the "Cesarean Variation" section in the description of each exercise, but realize that the timelines suggested will vary for individual cases. In general, the suggested timelines are on the conservative side. If you are fit going into surgery, your doctor may recommend some of the exercises even earlier than suggested.

---

*Baby Weight's* advising MD, Dr. Leighanne Glazener, OB/GYN at the Corpus Christi Womens Clinic in Corpus Christi, Texas, says: "I tell a new C-section patient on discharge that she can walk all she wants, but not to lift anything over 20 pounds for six weeks. She can drive when she can move well enough to comfortably turn and look over her shoulder and to stomp on the floor as is required to hit the car's brake quickly without hesitation, which is usually around the 2-week mark. I caution against any abdominal "crunch" exercises until 6 weeks post-op, when the fascial incision, the most important layer, is healed by at least 80%, to reduce the risk of hernia."

---

Your surgeon is familiar with your particular case and must ultimately be the one who clears you for exercise. You might be in a hurry to get moving and recover your shape, but returning to activity before your body is ready will result in a set back and slow your recuperation in the end. Sometimes even after you are medically cleared to exercise, you will feel discomfort during or after exercise, often felt as an uncomfortable pulling or burning sensation around the incision, or as an ache that lasts for several minutes or longer after activity. Heed the warning signs and reduce activity for a day or two. The best approach is to first listen to your doctor and then to listen to your body.

Your body might tell you it is okay to start moving, but you should only do so after your doctor tells you it's okay, too!

## Diastasis Recti and Exercise

During pregnancy, you should check yourself for diastasis recti at least once a week. A good practice is to begin every exercise session with the simple diagnostic maneuver outlined on pg. 47, for early detection of any change in the muscle separation. If you notice the gap between the muscles increasing but maintaining at less than 2 finger-widths, perform the Splinting technique described on pg. 90 with the other exercises to help prevent further separation. If the gap increases to more than 2 finger-widths, stop all supine exercises other than the isometrics (Pelvic Tilt and Activating Transverse Abdominus pg. 86-88) and the Splinting exercise (pg 90). You can perform up to 3 sets of 20 reps of those three exercises per session. It is safe to perform all the Seated Stretches exercises, as well as the Quadruped and Standing exercises. Plank should be performed only on the knees.

Postpartum, after a vaginal birth you can assess the gap on day 3. If you measure more than 3 finger-widths, perform only the isometric and Splinting exercises until the gap closes to less than 3 finger- widths, then include the other Beginner level exercises. After a C-section, wait until day 10 post-op to assess for diastasis recti, and start only the isometrics and Single Heel Slides. At 3 weeks post-op, reassess for diastasis and begin the Splinting exercise if necessary. Start the other Beginner exercises only after the gap is closed to 2 finger-widths and not before the time frame indicated in the Cesarean Variation section of each exercise, pending doctor approval, of course.

## CoreMama™ Terminology

**Sit bones-** The Ishia, the bones on which you sit.

**Pelvic Tilt-** Tucking the tailbone under to tilt the pelvis backward. While lying down, you maintain the pelvic tilt by pressing the low back flat and keeping it glued to the floor.

**Chest press-** Using your baby's weight in the postpartum program, press your baby up or out from your chest as you exhale, and draw the baby back in toward your chest as you inhale.

**Side Saddle-** Positioning the baby so that she is sitting on your hips or abdomen and facing the side, so that both feet are to the same side.

**Table Top-** Positioning the leg with the hip and knee bent to 90 degrees so the shin is parallel to the ground to form a flat, table-like surface while supine (face up). Double Table Top is the same but with both legs in Table Top position.

**Trembling is good-** Trembling is a sign of work, not weakness. When you tremble with exercise, you are challenging your body to its strength and endurance limits, which is the only way to get stronger. If it's easy, it is probably not doing much for you.

## Weight Bearing: Using Your Body Weight to Build Stronger Muscles and Bones

Walking, jogging, and pretty much anything done while standing is weight-bearing exercise. Weight-bearing exercise is extremely effective at muscle strengthening because it stimulates a co-contraction of opposing muscle groups all around a joint to stabilize the joint under the weight of the load. Weight-bearing exercise is the only form of exercise that causes bone growth. Bones adapt to the strain of weight bearing and muscle pull by generating more cells and becoming stronger. Practicing weight-bearing exercises regularly throughout pregnancy and for the rest of your life will help build and maintain bone strength, and will help prevent osteoporosis.

Even if you spend a great deal of your time on your feet, you still need to do weight-bearing exercises in order to build bone strength, because you must regularly increase the intensity and demand of weight bearing exercise to achieve the bone-building effect. Choose weight-bearing cardio activities to build cardiovascular endurance as well as muscle and bone strength, and regularly increase the intensity of the activities as you are able.

How much time do you spend per day taking weight through your hands and arms? Probably very little. The CoreMama™ program will teach you several upper extremity weight bearing exercises that help build muscle and bone strength in the arms and shoulder girdle as well. The CoreMama™ system gradually increases the intensity of a wide variety of upper extremity and lower extremity weight bearing exercises to maintain the muscle and bone-strengthening effects of the exercises. Since most people don't regularly bear weight through the wrists and hands, you may find those exercises uncomfortable at first. Try the modifications suggested in the individual exercises descriptions, and know that in just 3 to 5 sessions you will be stronger and accustomed to the new challenge.

# The CoreMama™ Exercises

The following exercises are specifically designed by a physical therapist and perinatal fitness educator to target the muscles most affected by pregnancy and childbirth. Strengthening exercises focus on the muscles that are overstretched and weakened, while specific stretches increase flexibility in those muscles that tend to tighten and bind. The result: counteracting the postural changes and resulting aches and pains that are common to nearly every pregnancy as well as preparing your body for and helping it recover from that awesome task of giving birth. CoreMama™ targets:

- The upper and mid-back extensors to diminish the hunchback effect
- The abdominals and low back extensors to stabilize the pelvis and lumbar spine and reduce the lumbar lordotic curve, thereby reducing low back pain and maintaining abdominal muscle tone
- The adductors and pelvic floor to focus on opening the pelvis for birthing, avoiding urinary incontinence in late pregnancy, and speeding the internal recovery after birth

The CoreMama™ program is based on principles of yoga, Pilates, and the general common sense approach of strengthening what is weak and stretching what is tight. The yogic philosophy of connecting with the breath and surrendering to strong sensation helps expectant mothers loosen tight muscles and connective tissue and establishes the body mind connection, which can help immensely during the childbirth and beyond. The core work derived from Pilates-type mat exercises focuses on strengthening the trunk stabilizers, reducing the risk of low back pain before and after giving birth and conditioning the muscles needed in the pushing stage of labor. A stronger core during pregnancy makes for a faster postpartum recovery of the waistline, guaranteed.

## USING YOUR BABY WEIGHT

Continue the CoreMama™ exercises *with* your baby after giving birth to rapidly re-coup your form, providing an opportunity to bond with your baby while taking care of yourself *and* maximizing the effects of the exercises by using the baby's weight for added resistance. The positioning and handling techniques used to incorporate your baby into the postnatal exercises, described under the "Using Your Baby Weight" heading of each exercise, help enhance your baby's gross motor development by facilitating greater head, neck, and trunk control. Mommy and baby grow stronger together by regular perfor-mance of these exercises.

## GETTING STARTED

Since the exercises indicated for expectant mothers are by and large the same exer-cises indicated for new mothers, they are presented together with a few modifications to accommodate for the obvious differences in the pregnant and postpartum body. Each exercise is described in detail with photos and special instructions for their prenatal and postnatal indications to avoid confusion. Exercises are grouped in sections by position, and presented in order of level of difficulty. The Beginner level is followed by the In-termediate and Advanced levels in each section. Additional postnatal exercises that are not appropriate during pregnancy are presented at the end of each section. Tune into BabyWeightTV™ to find a variety of CoreMama™ classes, from short beginner series to hour-long advanced level classes, at www.babyweight.tv.

You will need: a rug and/or yoga mat for padding, a towel to use as a prop, and your baby and/or a medicine ball for added resistance for the postpartum exercises. Review the different types of Kegel contractions on pg. 51, which are incorporated into many of the exercises. Unless otherwise indicated, start with 8 to 10 reps of each exercise and gradually increase to a full set of 20. Progress from one level to the next when you can easily do a full set of all exercises in that level.

## WARM UP AND COOL DOWN

It is important to ease the body gently into activity, especially the pregnant and postpartum body which undergoes dramatic changes daily. Starting every workout with a 3 – 5 minute warm up helps to loosen the muscles and tendons to avoid muscle strain or other injury. Finishing with a few minutes of cool down helps to release the lactic acid buildup in muscles which can cause muscle pain and soreness after exercise, and helps to gradually return the heart rate and muscle function to a resting state.

Recommended warm up activities: Start with one of the relaxation activities described below with Kegel exercises incorporated, then move gently into the sitting stretches featured on pg. 120 with special attention to connecting the movement with the breath. Follow with 3 or 4 of the Beginner level exercises, especially the Pelvic Tilt and Activating the Transverse Abdominus (pg. 86-88), and the Lunge Flow (pg. 148) to slowly increase the pace and intensity. Before cardio exercise, do a few sitting or standing stretches and start the activity itself at a slow pace for the first 3 to 5 minutes.

Recommended cool down activities: After a cardio activity, slow down but keep moving for a few minutes. Sitting Stretches and the Lunge Series at a very slow pace, always conscious of connecting the movement with the breath, are good ways to wind down after any exercise session. Finish with any of the relaxation techniques described below.

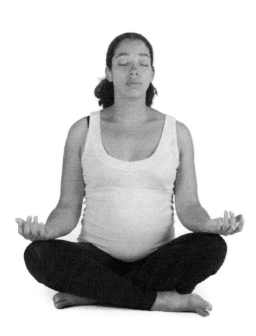

# Relaxation

You may not think of relaxation as exercise, but relaxing profoundly and regularly might even tie with Kegel contractions for the post of most important exercise in a prenatal and postpartum routine. While active exercises strengthen and lengthen the muscles that need it, conscious but passive relaxation helps alleviate physical and mental stress and connects you with your essence. Every exercise session, however long or short, should begin and end with some sort of relaxation exercise. Starting with a centering exercise sets the intention of establishing a connection with the body, getting *into* the body. This calming energy transmits to your baby, whether she is in the womb or in your arms.

## DEEP BREATHING

Find a comfortable position to sit on your exercise mat or rug, cross-legged with the sit bones up on a folded blanket or towel or up on a yoga block. Try traditional "Indian style" or place one folded leg in front of, rather than on top of, the other. If your hips are tight, place pillows under your thighs or knees for support.

Allow the eyes to close softly. Turn your focus inward; connect with your breath. In order to slow the breath, try to inhale to a count of six, hold the breath at the top for a count of six, and then exhale for the same count of six. Breathe deeply, focusing on the full rise of the inhalation and the complete fall of the exhalation. Visualize the breath starting deep in your belly, back behind your baby when you are pregnant, so that the belly expands first, then the ribs, chest, and collarbones follow. Once you establish the connection with the breath, visualize energy flowing up from the perineum through the central channel of the body, passing through the solar plexus, the heart, the throat, and out the top of the head. Engaging the pelvic floor muscles in a few gentle Kegel exercises as you inhale can help establish the connection with this energy flow.

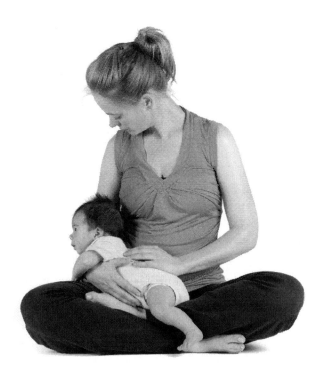

Time passes quickly once you get in touch with your breath. Without realizing it, you may pass several minutes here and feel profoundly relaxed and at peace when you come back to your physical body. It is most beneficial to practice this exercise on a daily basis, even several times a day.

## NECK ROLLS

Once you have established the connection with the breath and the energy, after several deep breaths, you can start to relax the parts of the body that tend to hold stress and tension. Inhale as you imagine a string pulling from the crown of the head up toward the sky to lengthen the spine. Exhale as you release the head forward, tucking the chin in toward the chest. On the next inhale, roll the chin toward one shoulder, feeling a great release in the opposite side of the neck, and exhale the head back to the center. Follow the rhythm of the breath, inhaling to the opposite side, exhaling to center. Repeat for 10 to 15 breaths. Finish by gently lifting the chin as you inhale. **Note**: You can do Shoulder and Neck Rolls in a variety of positions and situations, sitting in a chair in a waiting room or at your desk, sitting in a car at a stop light, standing in line at the grocery store. Just a few repetitions throughout the day can greatly reduce tension and stress in the neck and shoulders.

## Shoulder Rolls

Keep the connection with the breath. As you inhale, lift the shoulders up toward the ears. As you exhale, roll the shoulders down and back, the shoulder blades coming together toward the spine before gliding down the back in rhythm with the exhalation. Repeat for 10 to 15 breaths.

# Alternate Positions for Relaxation & Deep Breathing

## Child's Pose

This classic resting position derived from yoga is a lifesaver later in pregnancy when body aches and fatigue become more prevalent. After baby comes, it is great position to rest between exercises or just to relax. To get to child's pose, start in a hands and

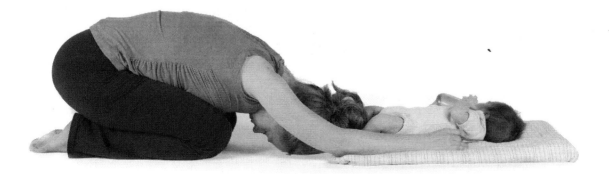

knees position with the knees wider than the hips to make space for a pregnant belly. Move the hips back to sit on the heels while the hands reach forward so the arms are outstretched. Try to rest the forehead on the floor. This position provides great relief for an achy back. It is also a fabulous place to do pelvic floor exercises, so while you rest the rest of you, do another Kegel or two!

## LEGS UP THE WALL

Start by sitting as close as you can to the wall, feet facing the wall. Use your hands to make your way to lying on your back and stretch the legs out straight with your feet up on the wall. Now scoot your rear even closer to the wall and consciously relax, releasing all tension from the shoulders and neck. You can place a bath towel folded in half then rolled lengthwise along the spine to help open the chest, and/or a folded blanket under the hips to facilitate a pelvic tilt. You should feel a gentle stretch in the backs of the thighs and behind the knees where the hamstring tendons pass. Pump your feet up and down and make circles in both directions with the feet to loosen the ankle joints and improve circulation. You can open the legs wide to feel the stretch more in the groin, or cross the ankles or place the soles of the feet together in a frog position to gently open the hips. Assuming this position for a few minutes two or three times throughout the day has a rejuvenating relaxation effect and also helps prevent varicose veins and swollen feet and ankles by improving lower extremity circulation. If you are more than 20 weeks pregnant and want to stay in this position for more than 3 to 5 minutes, place a flat pillow under one buttock to relieve pressure on the arteries that supply the uterus.

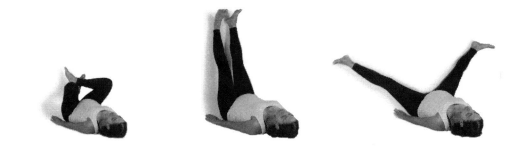

# Supine Series

Many effective core exercises are performed in supine, lying on your back. However, if you are more than 20 weeks pregnant, the supine position is not recommended for more than a few minutes at a time because the weight of the baby can occlude the arteries that provide the blood supply to the uterus. It is perfectly safe, though, to exercise in the supine position for the full term of your pregnancy if you change positions every 3 or 4 minutes. You should perform 3 or 4 of the supine exercises, then roll over to one side to perform the SideLying series, return to supine for 3 or 4 more exercises, roll to the opposite side for the SideLying exercises, and return to your back to finish the supine exercises. You can also alternate with the sitting, standing, and Quadruped (hands and knees) positions. After you have the baby, there is no such restriction, but the change of position might be just the distraction your baby needs to happily participate in your exercise plans.

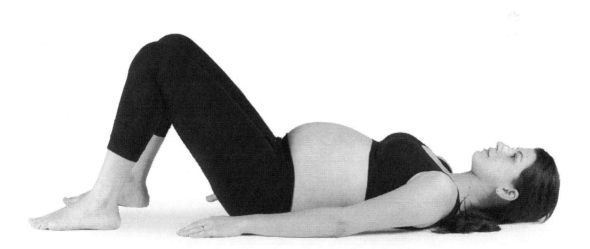

# Stretches On Your Back

It is important to rest and stretch in between abdominal exercises. The following stretches provide relief for a tight low back and help relax the core muscle groups.

# Hug your Knees

*The name describes it well. This gentle stretch works wonders on an achy low back.*

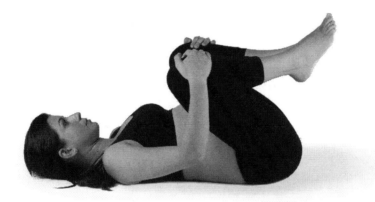

**Position:** Lying on your back with knees bent and drawn in toward the chest, on either side of your belly or your baby, as necessary.

**Action:** Breathe several deep breaths in the position, pulling the knees further in toward the chest each time you exhale. Gently rock your hips from side to side to deepen the relaxation. Add Slow Hold Kegel to this stretch, holding through several breaths. Repeat 3 to 5 times.

**Using your Baby Weight:** Position your baby on your chest. The relaxation will transmit to the baby through the close contact, the feel of your heartbeat, the gentle rocking motion, and the rhythm of your deep breathing.

**Cesarean Variation:** You can safely perform this exercise once your stitches are removed, letting pain be your guide to determine how far you push it.

# Happy Baby

*You will awaken your inner happy baby with this soothing stretch.*

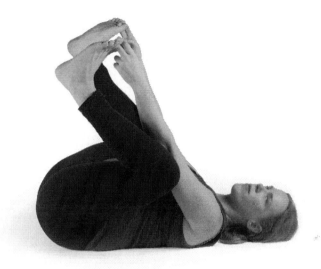

**Position:** Lying on your back with the Knees drawn in toward the chest.

**Action:** Take hold of both your big toes with the forefinger and middle finger and pull, drawing the knees in towards the armpits with the soles of the feet pointing upward toward the ceiling. Breathe deeply and gently rock side to side. Add the Elevator Kegel exercise to this stretch, holding the elevator at the top as you rock side to side for several breaths. Repeat 3 to 5 times.

**Using your Baby Weight:** Position your baby on your chest. Be careful not to get carried away and rock so far that you roll the baby off!

**Cesarean Variation:** You can safely perform this stretch once your stitches are removed as long as you don't' feel discomfort or pulling in the incision.

beginner level

# Activate Transverse Abdominus

*The horizontal fibers of this deep abdominal muscle form a waistband from the bottom of the ribs to the top of the pelvis. Maintaining and regaining tone in this muscle is essential in recovering the waistline after giving birth.*

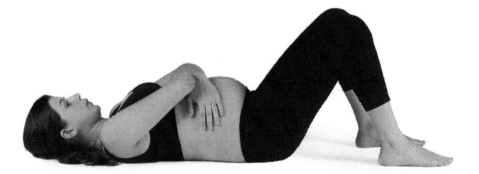

**Position:** Lying on your back with the knees bent and arms crossed over the belly with hands resting just below the ribs on either side.

**Action:** Inhale deeply through the nose, allowing the abdomen to rise and expand into the hands. Exhale slowly and completely through slightly pursed lips, feeling a strong tightening of the waistband with the fingertips. It often helps to make a long, slow "ah-hhhh" sound as you exhale. You should *not* lift your rear or "suck in" your belly. After a few reps, integrate a basic Kegel contraction as you exhale.

**Using your Baby Weight:** Rest your newborn on the pubic bone, her back supported by your thighs. A larger infant can sit upright.

**Cesarean Variation:** This exercise is safe to do as soon as day 10 after a C-section if your incision is closed and healing well. Position your baby on your chest to avoid pressure on the incision until 3 weeks post-op.

**Note:** After you get the hang of it lying on your back, try this exercise in other positions, such as hands-and-knees, sitting and standing. Like the pelvic floor, you can activate your transverse abdominus muscle anyplace, anytime. Coordinating it with an exhalation makes it most effective. Try it while rocking your baby in a rocking chair, rocking back as you exhale while contracting the transverse abdominus, inhaling to release as you rock forward.

# Pelvic Tilt

*This exercise is the basis of all exercises that follow. It is an isometric contraction of the entire abdominal brace with particular focus on the lower portion of the corset. Strengthen the core muscles while reversing the swayback curve inevitable to pregnancy.*

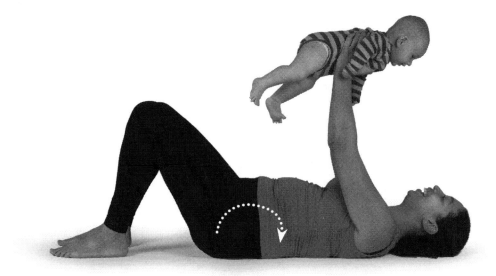

**Position:** Lying on your back with knees bent, hands resting by the sides, palms down. Note: try this exercise in other positions, such as hands-and-knees, sitting and standing.

**Action:** Inhale normally through the nose. Exhale slowly through the mouth, pressing the low back flat into the floor and drawing the bellybutton in toward the spine. Release as you inhale, repeat as you exhale for the first few reps. Progress to holding the tilt through a full breath before releasing. Add Fast Contract Kegel exercises as you exhale, progressing to the Slow Hold to hold the Kegel contraction while you hold the Pelvic Tilt.

**Using Your Baby Weight:** Rest your infant upright on your pelvis with her back resting on your thighs, supporting her with your hands if needed. Larger babies can sit upright. The baby's weight on your lower abdominals helps stimulate the contraction. Once you feel comfortable and competent with the pelvic tilt, you can hold your baby with straight arms up over your chest (as pictured) while you perform the set. She will love the flying sensation.

**Progression:** Even after you become advanced in the program, start every session with a set of 8 – 10 pelvic tilts to "wake up" the muscles and remind the body to maintain the pelvic tilt throughout the other exercises. If your program is limited due to diastasis recti or other conditions, perform up to 3 sets of 20 reps in a session.

**Cesarean variation:** This exercise is safe to do as early as day 10 after a C-section, though you may not feel comfortable having your baby anywhere near your incision until around 3 weeks post-op, in which case she can lie on her tummy on your chest.

# Splinting to Prevent or Correct Diastasis Recti

*This exercise is indicated in the event that your abdominal muscle separation approaches or exceeds 3 finger-widths. If you notice the separation increasing on your regular checks (see pg. 47) to two finger widths or more, follow the protocol outlined on pg. 75. Use this exercise to help close the gap postpartum before moving on to more advanced core exercises.*

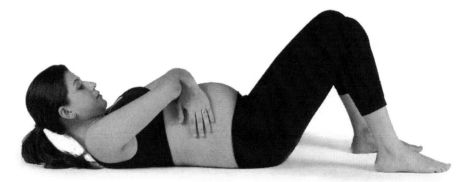

**Position:** Lying on your back with knees bent, arms crossed over the belly with one wrist above the other flat on your belly at level of the navel.

**Action:** Exhale slowly as you tuck your chin and lift your head while pressing gently inward with the hands and pulling the two sides of the rectus abdominus muscle toward the midline, closing the gap. Keep your shoulder blades on the floor.

**Using Your Baby Weight:** Place your newborn on your chest so you can kiss her as you lift your head. Her weight will help keep the upper body grounded.

**Progression:** Start with 10 reps 3 times a day, work up to 3 sets of 15 to 20 reps 2 to 3 times a day until the gap is closed to less than 2 finger-widths.

**Cesarean Variation:** Evaluate your rectus abdominus muscles at 3 weeks post-op and begin the Splinting exercise then if necessary.

# Single Heel Slides with Pelvic Tilt

*This exercise gently adds movement to the pelvic tilt stabilization.*

**Position:** Lying on your back with knees bent.

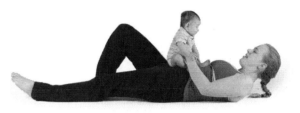

**Action:** Press your low back flat into the floor as you exhale. Hold the pelvic tilt as you slowly slide one heel away from your buttock, straightening the leg as you exhale, only to the point that you can still maintain the pelvic tilt. Bend the leg back in as you inhale, keeping the heel in contact with the surface at all times. Add a Slow Hold Kegel contraction as you exhale and hold it through the inhalation.

**Using Your Baby Weight:** Rest your infant upright on your chest or on your pelvis with her back resting on the nonmoving thigh, supporting her with your hands if needed. Larger babies can sit upright.

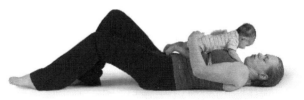

**Progression:** Tuck your chin to lift your head to activate the upper abs after you can easily do 20 reps with the head down. After you can do 20 reps without difficulty, eliminate this exercise and do instead the Double Heel Slide.

**Cesarean variation:** This exercise is safe to do as early as day 14 after a C-section with the head down and the baby on your chest to avoid pressure on the incision. Wait until 6 weeks post-op to try it with the head up.

# Double Heel Slide with Pelvic Tilt

*Increased challenge for the core muscles with simultaneous movement of both legs.*

**Position:** Lying on your back with your knees bent.

**Action:** Press your low back flat, then gently slide both heels away from the buttocks while exhaling, straightening the legs only so far as you can still maintain the low back flat on the floor. When you reach the point that the low back begins to arch, slowly inhale the legs back in *one at a time,* keeping the heels in contact with the floor and the low back pressed flat. Challenge your pelvic floor with a Kegel contraction as you exhale and hold it through the inhalation.

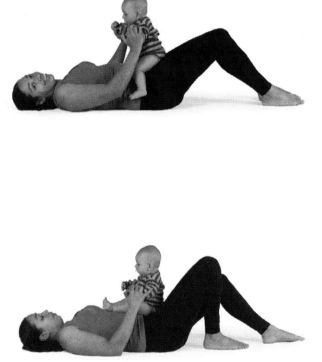

**Using your Baby Weight:** Rest your infant on your chest. Larger babies can sit upright on the pelvis, straddling or side-saddle. As you gain strength, you can hold your baby up above your chest.

**Progression:** When you can do 20 reps without difficulty, you are ready to begin the Pelvic Tilt in Double Table Top.

**Cesarean variation:** This exercise is safe to do as early as 3 weeks after a C-section if you are able to do 20 reps of Single Heel Slides without pain in the incision site.

# Single Knee Lifts with Pelvic Tilt

*Adds a more challenging against-gravity movement to the pelvic tilt stabilization.*

**Position:** Lying on your back with your knees bent

**Action:** Press your low back flat in a pelvic tilt, then slowly lift one knee as you inhale and lower the foot back down as you exhale. Always maintain a flattened low back. Repeat on the opposite side. Add Basic Kegel exercises, drawing in the perineum as you exhale and lower the leg, releasing as you inhale.

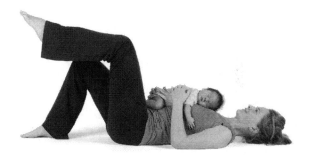

**Using Your Baby Weight:** Rest your infant on your chest. Larger babies can sit upright on the pelvis, straddling or side-saddle. Later, progress to holding the baby up over your chest and then to the Chest Press, pressing her up as you exhale and lowering her to the chest as you inhale.

**Progression:** After you can do 20 reps on each side without difficulty, eliminate this exercise and do instead the Toe Taps, but not before 6 weeks after a C-section.

**Cesarean variation:** This exercise is safe to do as early as 4 weeks after a C-section. Do not lift the baby with the exercise until 6 weeks post-op.

# Modified Single Leg Extension

*Stepping it up a notch with more difficult against-gravity movement.*

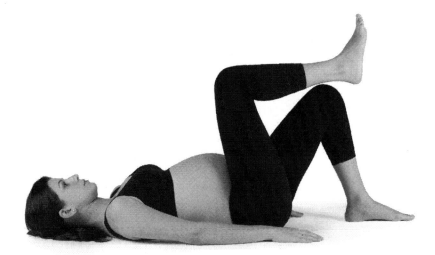

**Position:** Lying on your back with knees bent, one foot on the floor, the opposite leg in Table Top position with knee up and shin is parallel to the floor.

**Action:** Press low back flat into floor, activating the pelvic tilt. Inhale deeply, then extend the raised leg while exhaling, reaching out with the heel, keeping the low back glued to the floor. Inhale to bend the knee back to the Table Top position. The lower you extend the leg toward the floor, the more difficult it is to hold the pelvic tilt. Stay in control of the tilt! Add Kegel contractions as you exhale. Practice the Slow Hold through a few reps of this exercise.

**Using your Baby Weight:** Rest your infant upright on your pelvis with her back resting on the thigh of the leg with the foot planted on the ground, supporting her with your hands if needed. Larger babies can sit upright. The baby's weight helps stimulate the pelvic tilt. Later, progress to holding the baby overhead and the Chest Press.

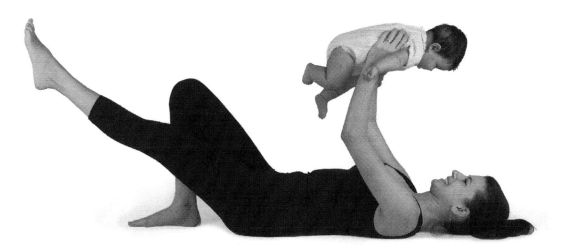

**Progression:** When you can do 20 reps with a strong pelvic tilt and without difficulty, begin also the Straight Leg Raise.

**Cesarean variation:** This exercise is safe to do as early as 4 weeks after a C-section if you can do 20 reps of Single Knee Lifts with control of the pelvic tilt and without pain. Don't hold the baby over your chest or do Chest Press until 6 weeks post-op.

# Straight Leg Raise

*Challenges the core while toning the thighs.*

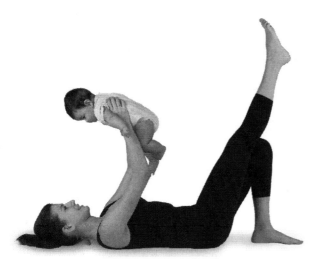

**Position:** Lying on your back with one knee bent and foot flat on the floor, opposite leg straight.

**Action:** Activate and hold the pelvic tilt, pressing the low back firmly into the floor. Lock the knee straight and lift the leg up to the height of the bent knee as you inhale. Exhale to lower the leg back down to *almost* touching the ground, hovering, while maintaining the pelvic tilt. Inhale to lift the leg up again, exhale to lower to hovering position just above floor. Keep your low back glued to the floor throughout the exercise. Add a Slow Hold Kegel contraction, working up to holding it through 5 reps or more.

**Using your Baby Weight:** Rest your infant upright on your pelvis with her back resting on the thigh of the leg with the foot planted on the ground, supporting her with your hands if needed. Larger babies can sit upright. The baby's weight helps stimulate the pelvic tilt. Later, hold your baby up over your chest for several reps or do the Chest Press, pressing up as you exhale.

**Cesarean variation:** This exercise is safe to do as early as 4 weeks after a C-section, but your doctor may want you to wait until 6 weeks post-op depending on your prior level of fitness and your individual circumstances. Even with doctor approval, only try this after you can do 20 reps of Modified Single Leg Extension without difficulty or discomfort. Don't hold your baby up or do the Chest press until 6 weeks post-op.

intermediate level

# Diagonal Cross Over

*This exercise activates the internal and external oblique abdominal muscles, which form the sides of the abdominal corset.*

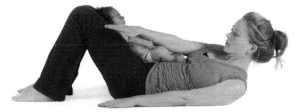

**Position:** Lying on your back with knees bent, feet hip-width apart, hands at sides.

**Action:** Press your low back flat in to the ground, activating and holding the pelvic tilt. On an exhale, tuck your chin in toward your chest while you reach across your body with your right hand, reaching outside the left knee so that the right shoulder moves forward and off the ground. Inhale yourself back down to the floor. Exhale to repeat on the opposite side.

**Using your Baby Weight:** Rest your baby on your thighs, either facing or away from you. Use your non-moving hand to stabilize the baby, staying on the same side for the full set instead of alternating. A larger baby can sit on your feet with her chest on your shins to help anchor your legs.

**Progression:** After you can do 10 reps without much difficulty, hold the contraction on the 5th rep while reaching across. Inhale deeply in that position, then pump the hand up and and down as if dribbling a small ball 7 times while exhaling. Repeat this variation again on every 5th rep as you increase to the full set of 20 reps.

**Cesarean Variation:** Wait until 8 weeks post-op to begin twisting-type exercises.

# Double Table Top Pelvic Tilt

*A more challenging position to perform the Pelvic Tilt.*

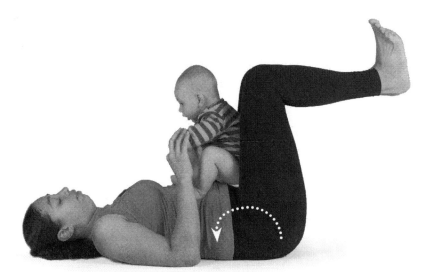

**Position:** Lying on your back with both hips and knees bent to 90 degrees, so that both shins are parallel to the floor to form a table-like surface in the Double Table Top position.

**Action:** Inhale deeply. Press your low back flat in a pelvic tilt as you exhale, holding the pelvic tilt through a full breath, relaxing on an inhalation. When you feel you have a strong pelvic tilt, add a Kegel contraction as you exhale.

**Progression:** After you can do 20 strong repetitions, progress to Toe Taps and Single Leg Extension from Double Table Top.

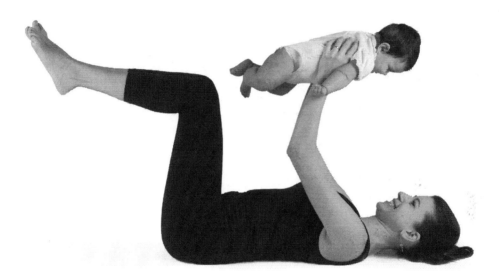

**Using your Baby Weight:** Rest your infant on your chest or upright on your pelvis with her back resting on the thighs, supporting her with your hands if needed. Progress to holding her up over your chest as you get stronger.

**Cesarean Variation:** Add this exercise at 5 weeks post-op only if you can perform 20 reps of Modified Single Leg Extension and Single Knee Lifts while maintaining a strong pelvic tilt. Assume the Double Table Top position by lifting *one knee at a time*. Add a folded towel under your hips to facilitate the pelvic tilt for the first week or so.

# The Fifty/Fifty

*This is a variation of the classic Pilates exercise "The Hundreds"; splitting the exercise into two parts makes it safe for the expectant and the new mother.*

*FIG. 1*

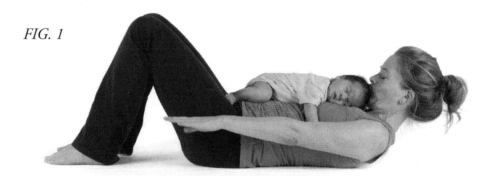

**Position 1:** Lying on your back with knees bent, feet flat on floor and hip-width apart, arms straight at sides with palms down (fig.1).

**Action 1:** Press the low back flat, tuck the chin, and lift the head, shoulders, and hands. Breathing continuously and deeply through the nose, gently pump the hands up and down just a few inches, as if you are dribbling two small balls. Try to breathe slowly to the count of five pumps as you inhale and five pumps as you exhale. Start with 5 deep breaths and work up to 10.

**Position 2:** Lying on your back with both knees up and shins parallel to the floor in the Double Table Top position (fig.2).

**Action 2:** Press the low back flat and lift the hands a few inches off the floor. Gently pump the hands while breathing deeply as described above, focusing on maintaining the low back glued to the floor. As you get stronger, practice straightening the legs up and out for a breath or two.

**Using Your Baby Weight:** Rest your infant upright on your pelvis with her back resting on your thighs or sitting upright for position 1. Shift the baby forward on the pelvis if she can sit on her own, or have her lying on the chest or pelvis for Position 2. Since your hands are busy pumping you won't be able to support her during this exercise.

**Postpartum Progression:** Once you are able to perform the Fifty/Fifty for 10 breaths in both positions, try performing the Full Hundred (described on pg.118).

**Cesarean Variation:** Practice only a modified version of Position 1 from 3 to 6 weeks post-op, keeping the head down on the floor or low pillow. At 6 weeks, you can lift the head and shoulder blades in position 1 and start Position 2, beginning w/ a folded towel under your hips to give your abs an advantage and help with the pelvic tilt.

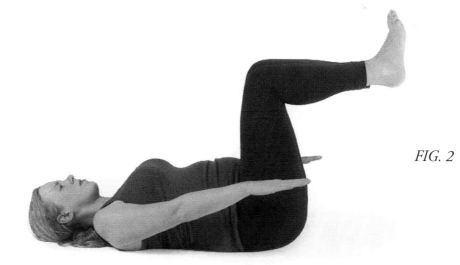

*FIG. 2*

# Toe Taps

*Challenging the core even more.*

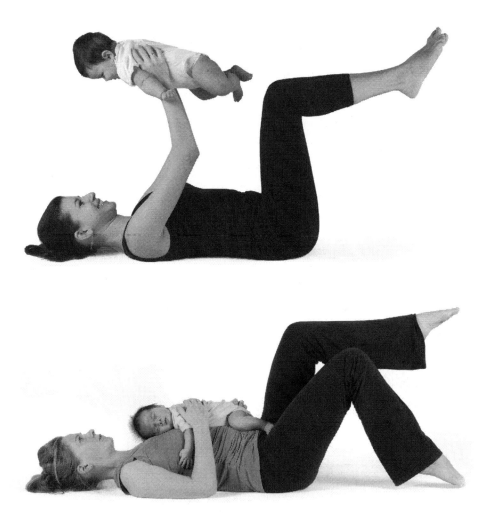

**Position:** Lying on your back with shins parallel to the floor in the Double Table Top position.

**Action:** Activate and hold the pelvic tilt. Inhale deeply through the nose, then, as you exhale, slowly lower one foot toward the ground to tap the toes, always pressing the low back flat into the floor. Inhale the leg back to Table Top position. Exhale to lower the opposite foot down to tap the toes. When you are able to do 5 on each side without much difficulty, add a Kegel contraction as you exhale and lower, relaxing it as you inhale and lift.

**Using Your Baby Weight:** Smaller babies can lie across your pelvis or chest. Larger babies can sit on the pelvis, side saddle or straddling. When you are strong enough to do 10 reps each side without great effort, you can hold your baby up over your chest throughout the exercise and later do the Chest Press, pressing the baby up as you exhale and lowering her down as you inhale. Start these variations for only 3 or 4 reps and increase gradually to the full set of 15 to 20 on each side.

**Postpartum Progression:** When you can do 15 reps on each side with out difficulty, try to do Double Toe Taps (pg. 114).

**Cesarean Variation:** Wait until at least 6 weeks post op to start this exercise, and only then if you are able to comfortably do 20 reps of the pelvic tilt in Double Table Top position, holding the contraction for one full breath each time. Start with 3 reps each side and work up to the full set of 20.

# Single Leg Extension from Double Table Top

**Position:** Lying on your back with both hips and knees bent to 90 degrees in the Double Table Top position.

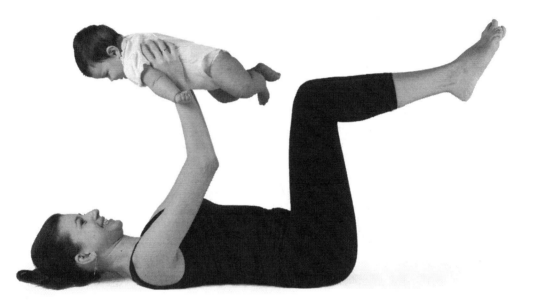

**Action:** Activate and hold the pelvic tilt. Inhale deeply through your nose, then exhale while straightening one leg, reaching up and out with your heel. The lower you take the leg, the more challenging for the abs. Only go as low as you can maintain the low back firmly glued to the floor. Inhale to bend the leg back into the Table Top position. Exhale to repeat on the opposite side. Practice Fast Contract and Slow Hold Kegel contractions through several reps.

**Using Your Baby Weight:** Smaller babies can lie across your pelvis or chest. Larger babies can sit on the pelvis, side saddle or straddling you. When you are strong enough to do 10 reps each side without great effort, you can step it up a notch and do the Chest

Press with your baby, lifting her up as you exhale and lowering her down as you inhale. Start this variation for only 3 or 4 reps and work your way up to the full set.

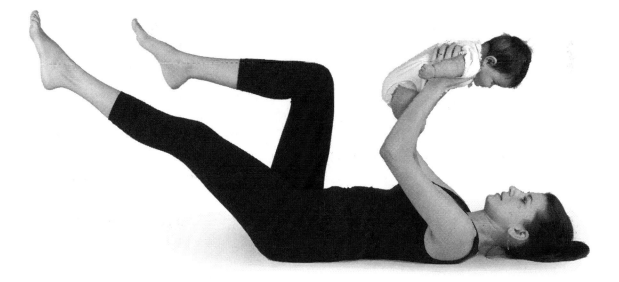

**Cesarean Variation:** Wait until at least 6 weeks post op to start this exercise, and only then if you are able to comfortably do 20 reps of the pelvic tilt in Double Table Top position, holding the contraction for one full breath each time. Start with 3 reps each side and work your way up from there to the recommended 20 for a full set.

# Bridging

*This exercise calls in the hip and back extensors to work with the abdominals for co-contraction of the core.*

**Position:** Lying on your back with the knees bent, feet flat on the floor and close to the seat.

**Action:** Inhale deeply through your nose. Exhale slowly while pushing through your feet to lift your rear as high as you comfortably can. Stay up through a full breath, long and slow. Slowly lower the hips back down to the floor as you inhale again, imagining lowering one vertebra at a time. After you can easily do 10-15 reps, practice staying up for 2 or more full breaths. Include the Elevator Kegel exercise as you exhale to lift your hips, holding it through the breaths at the top, releasing slowly as you lower the hips.

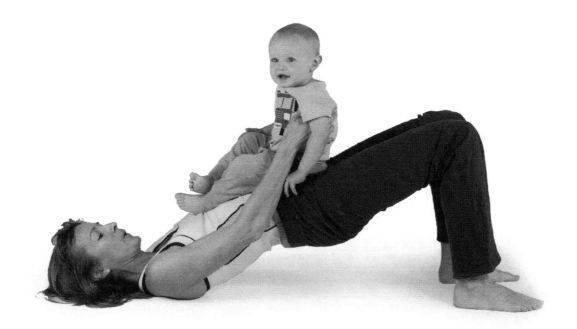

**Using Your Baby Weight:** Use your hands to support a smaller baby on your pelvis or chest. Larger babies can sit on the pelvis straddling you. The weight of the baby increases the challenge.

**Progression:** When you are strong enough to do 10 reps for 2 full breaths without great effort, add the Chest Press with your baby, lifting her over your chest as you exhale your hips up, holding her up through the full breaths, and lowering her down as you inhale the hips back down. Start this variation for only 3 or 4 reps and work your way up to the full set.

**Postpartum Progression:** When you can perform 10 reps of the bridge for 2 breaths each, you can try Extended Bridge on a stool or step (pg. 115).

**Cesarean Variation:** Wait until 6 weeks post op to start this exercise, limiting the height if you feel pulling or pain at the incision site.

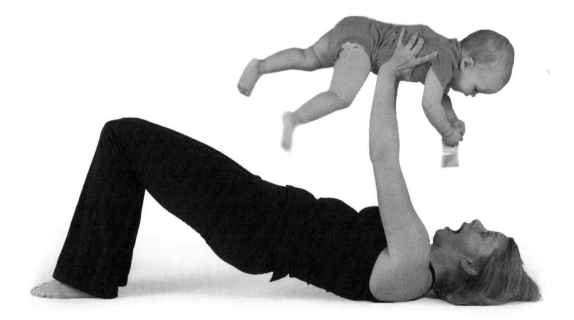

advanced

# Modified Hinge

*The weight of both legs straightening makes this exercise a real challenge.*

**Position:** Lying on your back with both hips and knees bent to 90 degrees in Double Table Top.

**Action:** Activate and hold the pelvic tilt. Inhale deeply through your nose, then, exhale to straighten both legs, reaching up and out with the heels. Only lower the legs as far as you can maintain the low back firmly glued to the floor. Inhale to bend the legs back into the Table Top position. You may find it more difficult to maintain the pelvic tilt after a few reps as you fatigue, in which case you should shorten the movement by reaching higher with the heels to complete the set. Trembling is good!

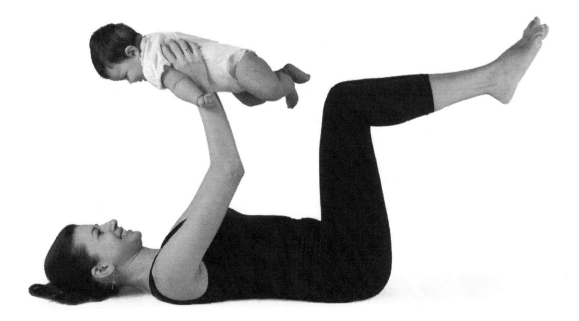

**Using Your Baby Weight:** Smaller babies can lie across your pelvis or chest. Larger babies can sit on the pelvis, side saddle or straddling you.

**Progression:** Start with 5 reps of this exercise. When you are able to do at least 10 reps without difficulty, try holding your baby up above your chest for a few breaths. The Chest Press is not recommended due to the concentration required to maintain the pelvic tilt in this position.

**Postpartum Progression:** When you can comfortably do 15 reps of the Modified Hinge, and no sooner than 8 weeks after having a C-section, you can begin The Hinge.

**Cesarean Variation:** Wait until at least 8 weeks post op to start this exercise, and only then if you are able to comfortably do 20 reps of the Toe Taps and Single Leg Extension exercises. Start with 5 reps and work your way up to a full set of 20.

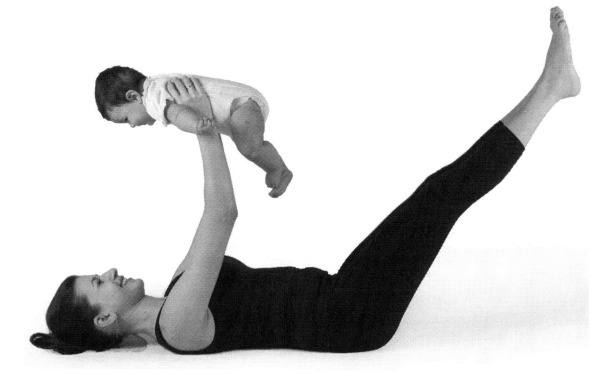

# Bicycle

*The simultaneous movement of both legs requires strength and coordination.*

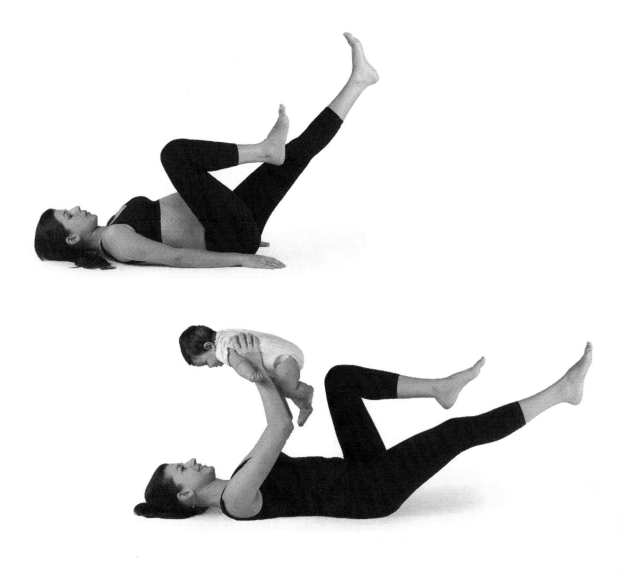

**Position:** Lying on your back with both hips and knees bent to 90 degrees in Double Table Top.

**Action:** Press the low back flat and inhale deeply. Exhale as you draw the right knee in toward the chest while reaching up and out with the left heel to extend the left leg. Inhale to begin to draw the left knee in toward the chest, then exhale as you complete the movement and fully extend the right leg. Keep the low back glued to the floor throughout the exercise. The lower you take the extended leg toward the ground, the more difficult. If you need to take the movement higher to maintain the pelvic tilt as you get tired, do so to complete the set.

**Using Your Baby Weight:** Smaller babies can lie across your pelvis or chest. Larger babies can sit side saddle or straddling your pelvis. When you are able to do a full set of 10 to 15 reps without difficulty, try holding your baby up above your chest for a few breaths. The Chest Press is not recommended due to the coordination required to synchronize the movement with the breath, and the concentration required to maintain the pelvic tilt.

**Cesarean Variation:** Wait until at least 8 weeks post op to start this exercise, and only then if you are able to comfortably do 20 reps of the Toe Taps and Single Leg Extension exercises. Start with 5 reps and work up to 20.

# Scissor Kicks

*Moving straight legs against gravity makes this the most difficult of the Supine Series exercises.*

**Position:** Lying on your back with both legs up straight as close to 90 degrees as possible while keeping the knees straight and toes pointed toward the ceiling.

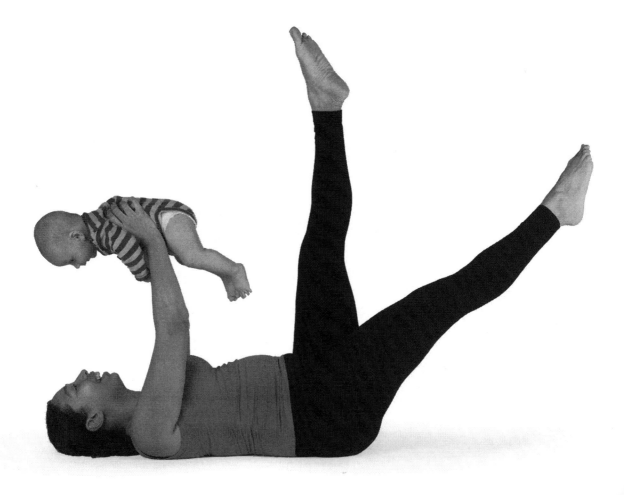

**Action:** Press your low back flat to activate the pelvic tilt. Inhale deeply through your nose, then slowly lower one leg down toward the ground as you exhale, only lowering the leg so far as you can maintain the low back glued to the floor. Inhale to lift the leg back up, exhale to lower the opposite leg. Keep the low back flat and both knees straight. As you get stronger, try taking the leg lower.

**Using Your Baby Weight:** Position your baby on your pelvis or your chest to help anchor your torso. When you are strong enough, try to hold your baby over your chest for a few reps at a time. The Chest Press is not recommended due to the strength and concentration required to maintain the pelvic tilt.

**Cesarean Variation:** Wait until at least 8 weeks post op to start this exercise, and only then if you are able to comfortably do at least 15 reps of the Toe Taps, Modified Hinge, and the Bicycle exercises. Start with 3 reps and work up to the full set of 20.

# Double Toe Taps

*Doubles the challenge for core stabilization.*

**Position:** Lying on your back with both hips and knees bent to 90 degrees in the Double Table Top position.

**Action:** Press the low back flat, then exhale slowly as you lower both legs to try to tap the toes. Only go so far as you can maintain the strong pelvic tilt. When you feel your back begin to arch, inhale to lift both legs back to Double Table Top. Start with 5 reps and work your way up to 20.

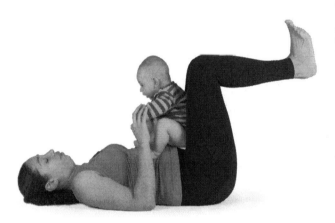

**Using Your Baby Weight:** Position your baby on your chest or pelvis to anchor your torso. After you can do 10 reps, hold her up overhead for a few reps at a time.

**Cesarean Variation:** Wait until 8 weeks to perform this exercise, and only after you can do at least 15 Toe Taps and Modified Hinge without discomfort.

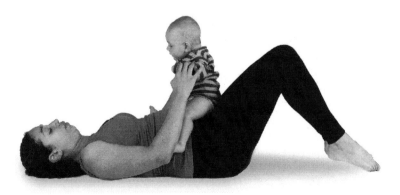

advanced – postpartum only

# Extended Bridge

*Begin the extended version of the Bridge on a stool or step only after you can perform 10 reps of Bridging without difficulty.*

**Position:** Lying on your back with both legs straight and feet up on a low stool or step.

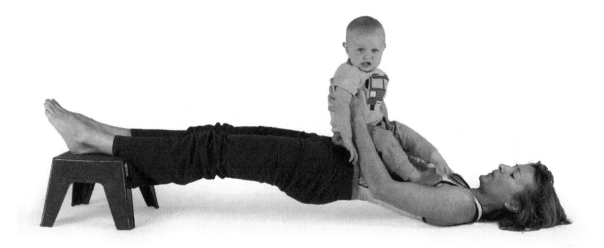

**Action:** Press through your heels to lift your rear as you exhale. Hold the contraction through a full breath before slowly lowering the hips as you inhale.

**Using Your Baby Weight:** Rest your baby on your chest. Larger babies can sit on your hips. Even toddlers love doing this exercise with mommy!

**Cesarean Variation:** Try this at 8 weeks post-op only if you are able to do 10 reps of the bridge without pain at the incision site.

# The Hinge

**Position:** Lying on your back with both legs straight, as near to 90 degrees as possible with the knees straight and reaching upward with both heels.

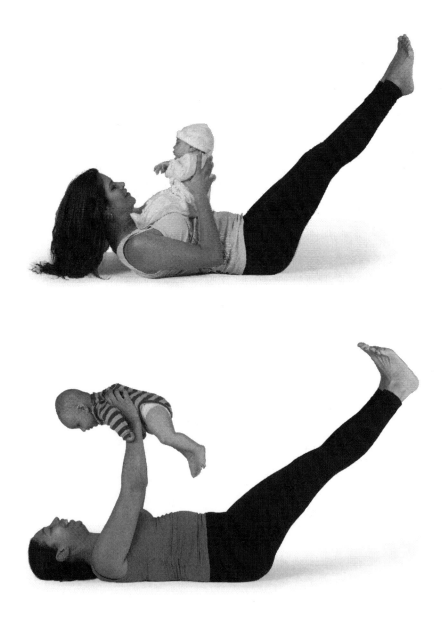

**Action:** Activate and hold the pelvic tilt then slowly lower the heels toward the floor while breathing deeply and continuously, keeping the low back glued to the floor. Take several breaths to lower the legs. Only go as low as you can maintain the flattened low back. When you feel your low back peeling up off the floor, bend your knees and start again. Add the Elevator Kegel exercises, holding the contraction at the top as you lower the legs down, releasing when you bend the knees. Remember, trembling is good!

**Using Your Baby Weight:** When you are able to do 10 reps, try holding your baby up above your chest for a few breaths. The Chest Press is not recommended.

**Progression:** Start with 3 reps, work up to 10. When you can comfortably do 5, try holding the legs at the height where you begin to lose the pelvic tilt for a full breath before bending the knees to start over. Also try to tuck your chin and lift your head and shoulders for one or more reps in a set, as pictured.

**Cesarean Variation:** You can try this at 8 weeks post-op if you can perform 20 reps of the Modified Hinge without pain at the incision site. Start with 3 reps and work your way up to 20, adding 3 reps at a time.

# Full Hundred

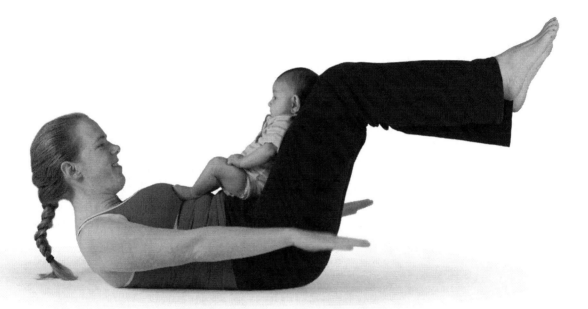

**Position:** Lying on your back with legs in Double Table Top position, press the low back flat and tuck your chin to lift the head, shoulders, and hands off the mat. Your neck and upper back should be rounded in a C-curve while you are looking at your navel.

**Action:** Inhale deeply through your nose as you begin to pump the hands gently up and down as if dribbling a small ball, inhaling to the count of 5 pumps, exhaling for 5 pumps. Start with 3 – 5 deep breaths, working your way up to 10 for the full hundred pumps (10 breaths at 10 pumps each). You can try to extend the legs to nearly straight for one or more breaths, being careful to always maintain the flattened low back. If you start to lose that pelvic tilt with straight legs, bend the knees to return to Double Table Top and continue to finish the set.

**Using Your Baby Weight:** Rest your baby on your chest for added resistance and some great snuggle time since you can kiss her when you lift your head. Larger babies can sit on your pelvis either side-saddled or straddling you, where the weight helps hold the pelvic tilt.

**Cesarean Variation:** Wait until 8 weeks post op to start this exercise, and only then after you can perform 10 reps each of the Fifty/Fifty exercise described on pg. 99.

***Note**: it is good to practice gentle neck stretches (see pg. 124) after this exercise in order to release all tension inadvertently held in the neck and shoulders.

# Sitting Series

## Seated Stretches

Practice these as warm-up or cool-down activities or as transitions between positions. Place your baby on a blanket or towel in front of you for these stretches, or position her on your legs to help anchor them. Repeat these and all stretches 3 to 5 times on each side.

## The Butterfly

**Position:** Seated with soles of the feet together in front and drawn in close to the groin, hands resting on the feet.

**Action:** As you inhale, imagine a string pulling you from the crown of your head upward as your spine grows longer. As you exhale, gently press the knees closer to the floor. Don't bounce! Ease gently into the stretch. You should feel this stretch deep in the hips and groin. If you have the flexibility, you may try to walk your hands forward to deepen the stretch. Stay in the stretch for at least 5 deep breaths. Add an Elevator Kegel exercise, holding the Elevator at the top through the several deep breaths while down in the stretch.

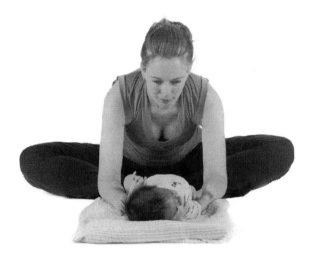

# Wide Leg Stretch

**Position:** Seated with legs open wide, knees straight, toes pointed up toward the ceiling.

**Action:** Inhale to grow the spine longer, exhale as you walk the hands forward, keeping a straight spine. Stay for several deep breaths, deepening the stretch as you exhale. Do not bounce! You should feel this stretch on the backs of the thighs and in the groin and inner thighs. Once you are as deep as you can go in the stretch, practice alternating Fast Contracts with Slow Hold Kegel exercises.

**\*Note:** If you have pubic symphysis pain, avoid this stretch and do instead the Side Leg Stretch with one leg bent.

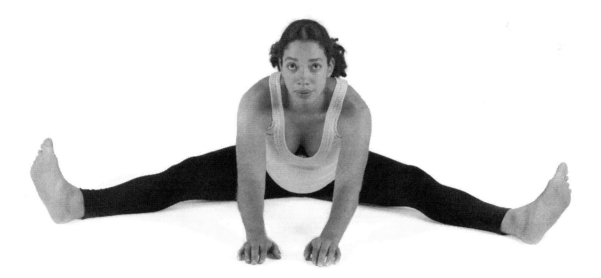

# Side Leg Stretch

**Position:** Sitting with one leg bent and the foot close to the groin, the opposite leg straight with toes pointing upward.

**Action:** Inhale to a longer spine while reaching upward with the hand on the same side as the bent leg, exhale to slide the other hand down the straight leg as the upper arm reaches up and over. Draw the upper shoulder back. If you are able, place the lower elbow on the floor inside the knee and reach over toward your foot with the upper hand, taking care to always pull back with the shoulder. Breathe several breaths, trying to deepen the stretch gently each time you exhale. Try to hold the stretch for 10 breaths while doing 10 Kegel contractions.

**Cesarean Variation:** Do this without reaching up with the arm until 4 weeks post-op, to avoid unnecessary pulling at the incision site.

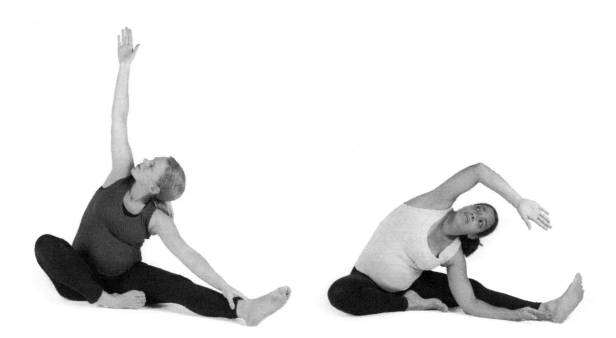

# Neck and Shoulder Stretches

These stretches are a lifesaver for the pre- and postpartum period and beyond. You will soon appreciate how this release can profoundly reduce tension held in the neck and shoulders. You can do them anywhere… sitting at your desk, in line at the grocery store, or waiting at a traffic light.

**Position:** Sitting with legs crossed or in the Butterfly position.

**Cesarean Variation:** Wait until 2 weeks post-op to do upper extremity stretches to avoid strain on the incision. You can practice the neck stretches from day 1 post-op.

# Triceps Stretch

Reach up overhead with one hand as you inhale, then bend that elbow to place the hand between your shoulder blades. Place the opposite hand on the upper elbow and draw it closer to your head. You should feel the stretch in the back of the upper arm and along the side of the body. Avoid pushing your head forward. Hold for 10 deep breaths before repeating on the opposite side. Add an Elevator Kegel contraction to this stretch, holding it at the top for several breaths.

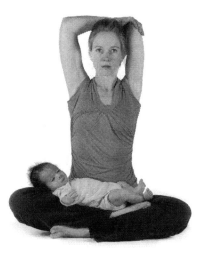

# Shoulder Rotator Stretch

Reach upward with one arm as you inhale, and place that hand between your shoulder blades as you exhale. Take the other arm back behind your back so that the back of the hand is resting on the back, reaching for or grasping the opposite hand (fig. 1). If you don't reach the hand, just take hold of your shirt with both hands and enjoy the stretch. You can hold a towel or a belt in your hands to maximize the stretch by *gently* pushing upward with the upper hand or pulling downward with the lower hand. You should feel this deeply in both shoulders. Hold for 10 deep breaths before repeating on the opposite side.

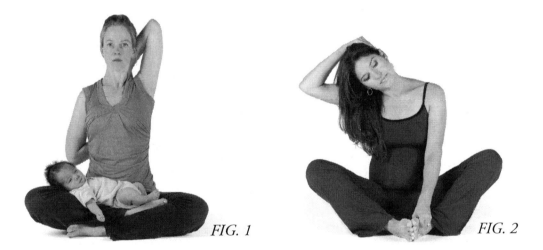

*FIG. 1*                                                                                    *FIG. 2*

# Cervical Release

Begin by imagining a string pulling you from the crown of your head upward as you inhale, lengthening the spine. As you exhale, drop the right ear toward the right shoulder to release the left side of the neck. Gently rest the right hand on the left ear, allowing gravity to deepen the stretch (fig. 2). Important: do not pull! Hold the stretch for a 3-5 deep breaths. Release the hand from the head and return the head to center as you inhale, then exhale to repeat the stretch on the opposite side.

Perform the same stretch *forward* to release the neck extensors by dropping the chin toward the chest as you exhale, resting a hand on the back of the head. Hold for several breaths.

# Core Rowing

*Stretches the hamstrings while mobilizing the pelvis and working the abs.*

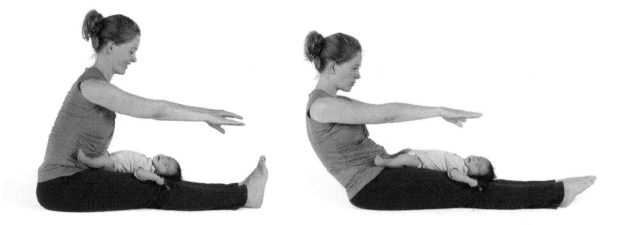

**Position:** Sitting with a long spine with your legs in front of you, feet flexed back toward you. Arms straight out in front at shoulder height. It helps to move the flesh to connect the sit bones to the ground before starting this exercise, by lifting each buttock upward from behind.

**Action:** Inhale deeply through the nose while you reach forward toward your toes, trying to keep your back straight. Exhale to roll back to sit onto your sacrum. Inhale back up to sit high on the sit bones and reach the hands forward toward the toes, exhale to roll back. Practice Fast Contract Kegel contractions as you exhale and roll back, releasing as you inhale forward.

**Using Your Baby Weight:** Position your baby in sitting or lying down on your shins or thighs to help anchor your legs.

**Cesarean Variation:** Wait until 6 weeks post-op to start this exercise. If you experience pain or a pulling sensation at the incision site, try shortening the movement to not roll back so far.

# Pelvic Rocking

*This exercise explores the full range of motion of the pelvis and helps to reverse the swayback curve common to pregnancy.*

**Position:** Sitting high on the sit bones, with knees bent and feet flat, hands on out sides of thighs close to the knee.

**Action:** Imagine a string pulling you up from your chest toward the ceiling to open your heart toward the sky as you inhale deeply through the nose. Exhale slowly as you hollow out the abdomen, rolling back to sit on the sacrum. Try to keep the shoulders back to avoid rounding too much in the upper back, isolating the movement to the pelvis. Inhale yourself back up to sitting high on the sit bones, imagining that string pulling you from the sternum up toward the ceiling. Don't use your hands to pull yourself up.

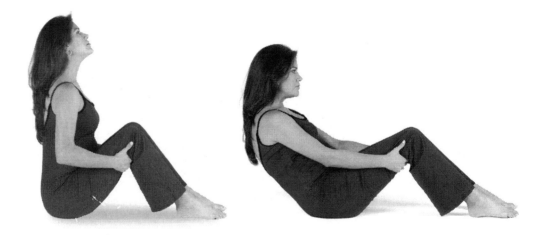

**Using Your Baby Weight:** Place your baby on your thighs, facing you. You can make conversation with her, especially as you roll back, to help you remember to exhale and not to hold your breath. Another option: place a bigger baby's belly on your shins with her arms over your knees, using your hands to stabilize her or to hold her hands gently. Later try doing the Chest Press with your baby, pressing her out away from your chest as you exhale and roll back, as pictured below.

**Postpartum Progression:** When you are able to do 10 reps of Pelvic Rocking without difficulty, and not before 8 weeks after a C-section, you can try The Boat.

**Cesarean Variation:** Wait until 6 weeks post op to start this exercise.

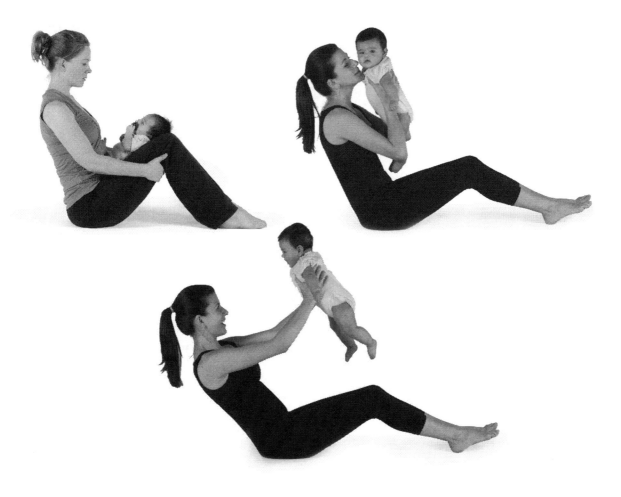

intermediate – postpartum only

# The Boat

*A core-engaging challenge for the Postpartum Mom. Baby will love this and you will too!*

**Position:** Sitting with a straight spine and bent knees, beginning with feet on the floor and hands behind the thighs or supporting your baby.

**Action:** Use your hands to help draw the knees in toward your chest while you lift the

feet to balance on the sit bones. Lift the feet to make the shins parallel to the floor. Keep your shoulders back to keep the heart open as you release your hands from behind the thighs, keeping your shins parallel to the floor. Breathe at least 3 deeps breaths in the position; work your way up to 5.

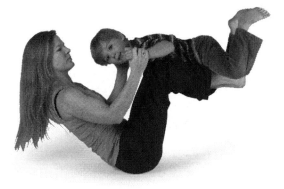

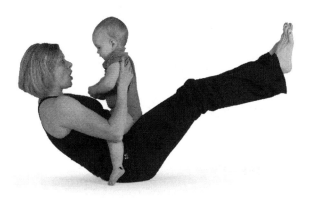

**Using Your Baby Weight:** Place a small infant on your pelvis with her back to your thighs. A larger baby can sit upright on the pelvis or on your feet with her chest to your shins while you hold her hands. You can practice this with very big babies if you have the strength! Leave your baby on your pelvis to practice the more advanced straight-leg version.

**Progression:** Start with 3 reps for 3 breaths with bent knees, working your way up to 10 reps for 5 breaths. After you can do 5 reps for 5 breaths, lift the feet to straighten the legs as much as possible before releasing the handhold and keep the height in the legs as you breathe 3 to 5 deep breaths. Remember, trembling is good!

**Cesarean Variation:** At 6 weeks post-op you can try a modified version of the Boat by balancing on the sit bones and continuing to hold behind the thighs (not releasing the hand hold), or by keeping the feet on the floor and reaching upward with the hands as you lean back, keeping an open heart and a straight spine. Try the full version of the Boat at 8 weeks post-op if you can easily do 5 reps for 5 breaths of the modified versions. Add the baby's weight only after you can do 5 reps of the full Boat without discomfort.

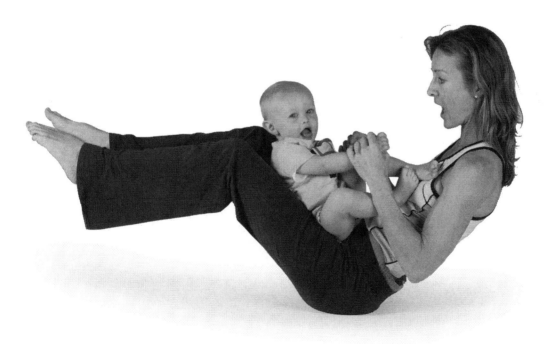

# SideLying Series

It is important to change positions frequently, especially while performing exercises on your back when pregnant. Moving to your side relieves pressure from the weight of the uterus and allows you to work your hip muscles against gravity. It is a good practice to roll to one side to exercise or to rest after doing 2 or 3 of the exercises on your back, then return to your back to do a few more exercises before moving to the other side. Once you have the baby, there is no such restriction but the change of position is still good for variability so that neither mommy nor baby get bored.

**Using Your Baby Weight:** Place your baby on her back or her belly on a folded towel in front of you at shoulder-level for these exercises. She will enjoy the face-to-face interaction and the tickles you can deliver in this position. You can give her tummy time here too, encouraging her to lift her head to watch your show.

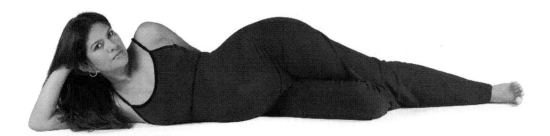

# Hip Abduction (Side Leg Lifts)

*Trims the saddle bags for firmer thighs.*

**Position:** Lying on your side with the bottom leg bent and the top leg straight and in line with your body, propped on your elbow, cradling your head in your hand.

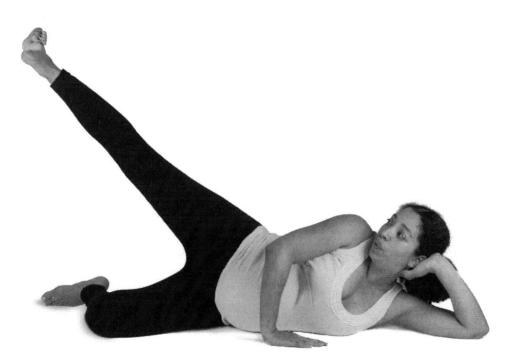

**Action:** Inhale deeply through your nose. Exhale slowly as you lift your straight leg toward the ceiling, with foot flexed and toes pointed straight ahead, knee locked straight. Inhale as you lower the leg to hover above the opposite leg, not touching. Draw the navel in toward the spine to keep the torso stable throughout the exercise. Repeat for 10 reps in rhythm with your breath, exhaling as you lift and inhaling as you lower the leg.

Finish with a straight leg stretch up to side, bending the knee in to take hold of the big toe with two fingers before straightening the leg as in figure 2. Hold the stretch for 5 deep breaths before releasing slowly. Add Fast Contract Kegel exercises, contracting with the leg lift as you exhale, releasing as you inhale and lower the leg.

**Cesarean Variation:** At 3 weeks post-op you may be able start with a few reps in a limited range (only lifting about halfway) if it feels comfortable. Stop and wait a while longer if you experience any discomfort in the incision with the exercise.

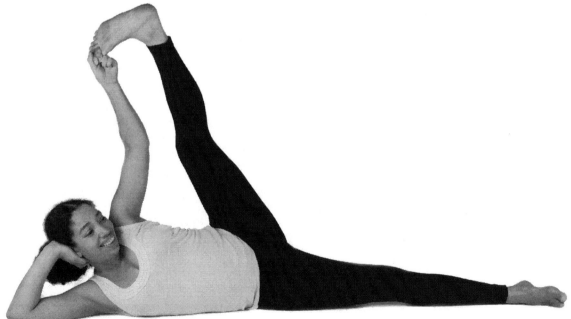

*FIG. 2*

# Hip Adduction (Inner Leg Lifts)

*Works the inner thigh to smooth unwanted curves.*

**Position:** Lying on your side with the top leg bent and foot placed in front of you, holding the ankle with the top hand to stabilize the foot. Lock the bottom leg straight in line with the body with the toes pointing forward.

**Action:** Inhale deeply through your nose. Exhale slowly as you lift your bottom leg straight up, with the knee locked straight and toes pointed straight ahead. Repeat for 10 reps in rhythm with your breath, exhaling as you lift and inhaling as you lower the leg. Practice Fast Contract Kegel exercises with this, contracting in the perineum as you lift the leg, relaxing as you lower it.

**Progression:** Work up to 2 sets of 10 reps of each of the two Leg Lifts, one after another or broken up into 2 rounds of the whole SideLying Series mixed in with the Supine Series.

**Cesarean Variation:** Wait until 4 weeks post-op to begin this exercise, if you feel comfortable getting into the position and have no pain in the incision with the leg lift.

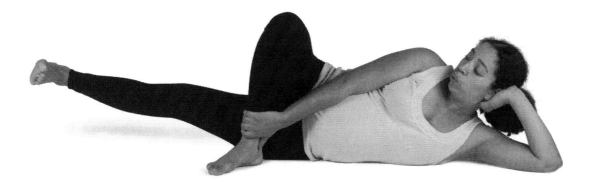

# Hip Dips

*A great upper body weight-bearing exercise that fully engages the core, a tough exercise that is safe for all levels.*

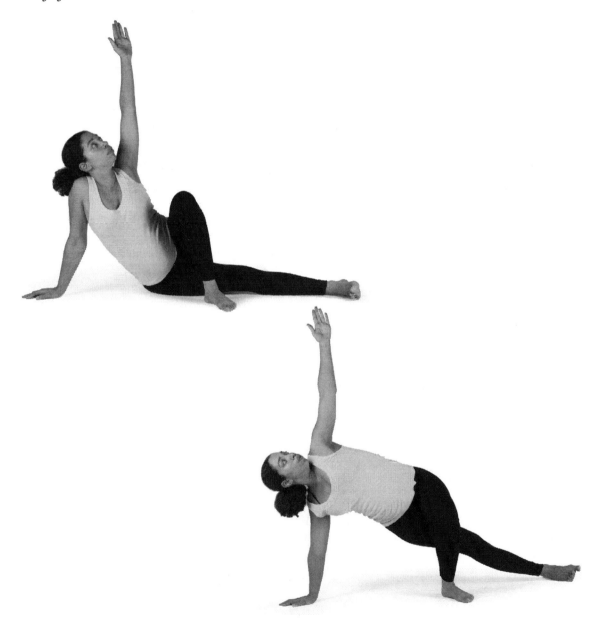

**Position:** Lying on your side with the top leg bent and foot flat in front of you, bottom leg straight and in line with the body with toes pointed straight ahead (the same position as for the Inner Leg Lift).

**Action:** Press up onto the bottom hand to extend the arm with fingers pointed away from the hip. Reach toward the ceiling with the top hand and inhale deeply. Exhale slowly as you press into the flat foot to lift your hips toward the ceiling, weight-bearing through the outer edge of the bottom foot. Imagine a sling under your hips pulling them upward. Inhale as you slowly lower back to the floor, looking down toward the bottom hand. Continue in rhythm with your breath, exhaling to lift the hips and inhaling to lower the hips. Include Fast Contract and then Slow Hold Kegel exercises, contracting as you exhale up, relaxing as you inhale down.

**Progression:** Start with 3 – 5 reps and work your way up to 10 on each side. After you can easily do 10 reps, try maintaining the position at the top (hips raised) for a full breath before lowering down, starting again with 5 reps.
**Postpartum Progression:** After you can perform 10 Hip Dips, holding for a full breath, try the Side Plank (pg. 136).

**Cesarean Variation:** Wait until 6 weeks post-op to start this exercise. If you feel pain in the incision, wait another week.

advanced – postpartum only

# Side Plank

**Position:** From the Hip Dips position, while the hips are up in line with the body, place your top foot just in front of the bottom foot. Or from the Plank, move one hand directly under your nose and roll over to the edges of your feet as you lift the opposite hand up toward the sky. If the weight bearing hurts your wrist or if you have a history of carpal tunnel syndrom, try it down on your elbow.

**Action:** Hold for a full breath, imagining a sling pulling your hips upward, before lowering the hips or rolling back over to the Plank. Remember, trembling is good!

**Progression:** Gradually work your way up to 5 breaths for 5 – 10 reps. Increase the difficulty later by stacking the top foot on top of the lower foot (fig. 2).

**Cesarean Variation:** Start Side Plank at 8 weeks post-op if you can do 10 reps of Hip Dips, held for a full breath at the top, and as long as you have no discomfort.

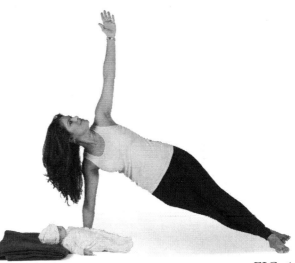

*FIG. 1*

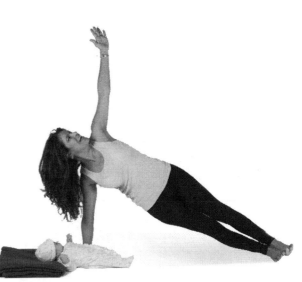

*FIG. 2*

# Quadruped Series

*The hands and knees position allows full range of motion of the pelvis and encourages co-contraction of the entire core. You can perform the Beginner Level Quadruped exercises even in the event of diastasis recti.*

**Position:** Alignment is easy – just place your hands directly beneath your shoulders and your knees directly below the hips.

**Cesarean Variation:** You can start most of the Beginner level exercises at 4 weeks post-op, if your doctor approves and you have no discomfort in the incision. Wait 8 weeks to try Thread the Needle to avoid too much pull on the scar in its most fragile time.

**Using Your Baby Weight:** Position your baby on a folded towel or blanket under your face to have a comical interaction as you perform the following exercises.

**Note:** If you have wrist pain or a history of carpal tunnel syndrome, place your hands further forward to reduce the angle of wrist extension, or make fists and assume the position up on your knuckles.

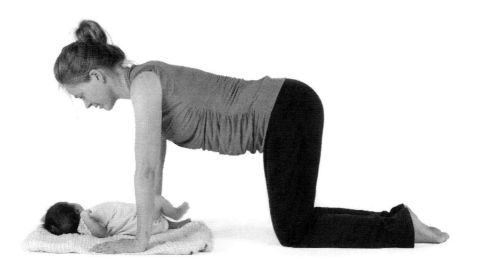

# Abdominal Bracing

*Activating the transverse abdominus muscle*

**Action:** with a neutral spine (flat back), practice contracting the transverse abdominus muscles on an exhale as described on pg. 86. You should feel a tightening all around the abdomen, including in the sides. Do at least 5 repetitions to awaken the abdominal corset before continuing with the other quadruped exercises.

# Pelvic Rocking

*As the name indicates, the movement is focused in the pelvis.*

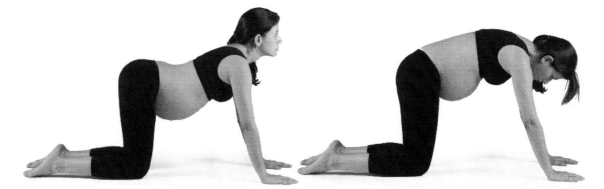

**Action:** As you inhale through your nose, lift your tailbone up toward the ceiling while you lift your chin and allow your chest to sink down toward the floor so that the shoulder blades come together. Exhale to tuck the tailbone under and bring the chin back down to neutral so that you are looking at the place between your hands and your neck is straight, *not* rounding the upper back so as not to encourage the hunchback curve. Continue in rhythm with your breath, inhaling to lift the tail and drop the chest, exhaling to tuck the tail. Repeat for 10 reps.

# Tail Wagging

*Works the sides of the abdominal corset and loosens the lumbar spine.*

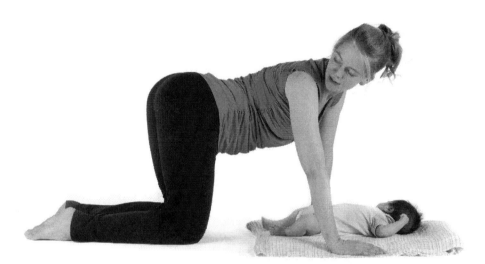

**Action:** With a neutral (straight) spine, inhale deeply through the nose then exhale slowly as you look over one shoulder toward your hip, moving the shoulder toward the hip and the hip toward the shoulder. Inhale back to the neutral position. Exhale to the opposite side. Try to keep equal weight in both hands and draw the navel in toward the spine throughout the entire exercise. Repeat for 10 reps on each side.

# Thread the Needle

*Mobilizes the mid back and reverses the hunchback curve, ends with a welcome rest and a divine thoracic stretch.*

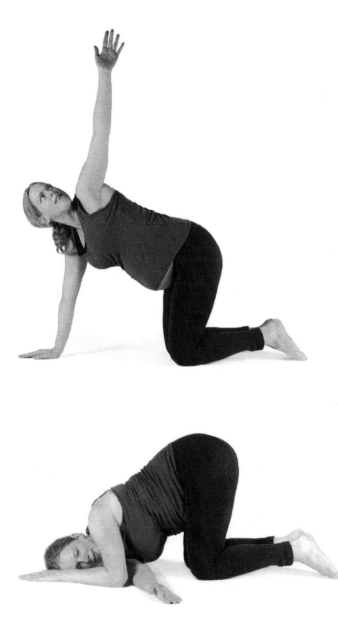

**Action:** From a neutral position, draw the navel in toward the spine and inhale one hand out to the side and up toward the ceiling to open the shoulder as you look upward toward the hand. Exhale the hand back down to the mat. Repeat on the opposite side on the next inhale. On the 5th breath on each side, take the hand through the space between the opposite arm and leg as you exhale, bending the supporting elbow to allow you to lower your ear down to the ground. You should feel a stretch behind your shoulder blade. Stay there for 10 deep breaths.

Practice the Elevator Kegel exercise while in the stretch. Use the energy of an inhalation to help you rise back up to hands and knees to finish with one last twist and the stretch on the other side.

intermediate level

Include these exercises after you can perform 10 reps each of Pelvic Rocking and Tail Wagging without difficulty.

# Fire Hydrant

*Strong work in the hips and core helps combat flabby thighs and not-so-lovely love handles.*
**Action:** With a neutral spine, draw the navel in toward the spine as you inhale deeply

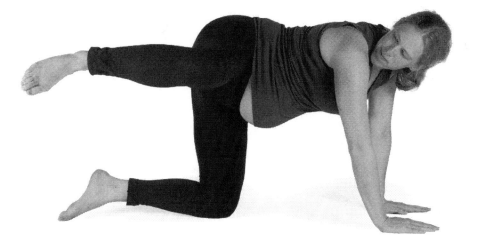

through the nose, shifting your weight to your right knee. Exhale to lift the left leg up to the side with the knee bent and look toward the knee. Inhale the leg back down toward the floor but not touching the floor, turning your gaze back down to between your hands. Exhale the leg back up, looking at the knee. Inhale it back down. Repeat for a total of 5 breaths on the same side. On the 5th repetition, when the leg is up, extend the leg straight to the side and look at the foot, trying to keep the leg at hip height (fig. 2). Try to hold the leg outstretched for a full breath before bending it and lowering it back to the floor. Shift the weight to the left and repeat on the right leg. As you become stronger, you can challenge yourself more by trying to hold the leg outstretched for up to 5 breaths. Later still, you can do 2 sets of 5 on each side.

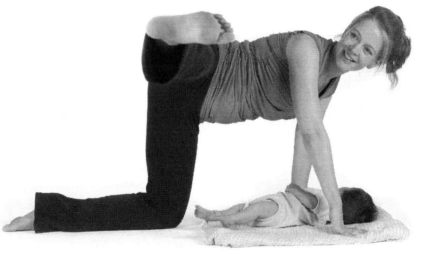

*FIG. 2*

**Cesarean Variation:** Wait until 8 weeks post-op to attempt the Fire Hydrant, eliminating the leg extension on the 5th rep for the first week. Add the leg extension only if you don't feel any discomfort at the incision site.

# Bird Dog

*Maximum co-contraction of the entire core in this balance-challenging pose.*

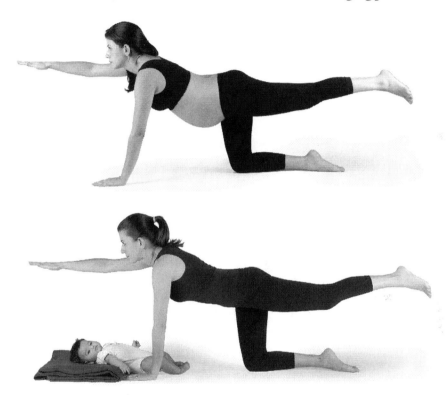

**Action:** With a neutral spine, exhale to lift one leg out behind you to make it parallel with the ground. Focus on a point on the floor about a meter out in front of you. After you find your balance, lift the opposite hand to stretch the arm out in front (like a bird dog points when it hunts). Think length not height, only taking the arm and the leg up to the point that they are parallel with the ground. Breathe slow and continuous breaths, drawing the navel in toward the spine to stabilize the pose. Start with 2 to 3 breaths and work your way up to 5. Repeat at least 2 reps each side, working up to 5 as you are able.

**Cesarean Variation:** Wait until 8 weeks post-op to attempt this exercise, and only lifting the leg for the first week or so. Then add the arm movement if you don't feel any discomfort in the area of the incision.

# Floor Series

Mix these exercises into your routine as you move from quadruped and sitting positions to practice one or more of the following exercises at a time.

## Downward Facing Dog (Hiking a Leg)

*This exercise combines an all-over stretch with full body strengthening.*

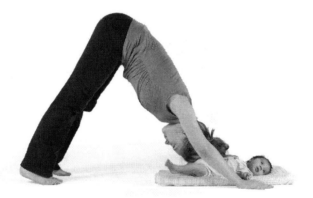

**Position:** From hands and knees position, tuck your toes under and straighten your legs to lift your hips. Hands are shoulder-width apart. Feet are hip-width apart.

**Action:** Breathe several deep breaths in this position as you try to lengthen the spine by rotating the sit-bones up toward the ceiling. You can alternate bending one knee, allowing the opposite heel to move closer to the floor, for a few breaths before trying to take both heels closer to the floor. Press firmly into the floor with the hands, especially with the thumb and forefinger. Breathe deeply and continuously through your nose. After several breaths, slowly lower down to rest on hands and knees or sit back in to Child's

Pose (see pg. 81). Start with 3 repetitions for 5 breaths. Work your way up to 5 reps of 8 – 10 breaths. The repetitions don't have to be consecutive. Mix it in with the other exercises in the Floor Series or the Quadruped Series.

**Progression:** When you can comfortably do 5 reps of the static position for 5 breaths, you can begin to practice Leg Lifts (Hiking a Leg) in the same position. Simply shift your weight to one foot while you lift the opposite leg up behind you, opening the hip to stack the top hip directly on top of the other, as you inhale. Try to keep weight bearing equal in both hands. At first just inhale the leg up and exhale it down. As you get stronger, hold the leg up for a full breath before lowering.

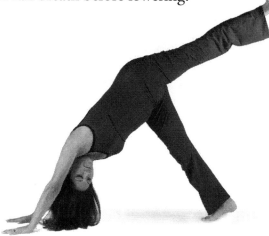

**Postpartum Progression:** When you can do 5 reps of the Downward Facing Dog Hiking a Leg without difficulty, progress to the Flying Pigeon Flow.

**Using Your Baby Weight:** Have your baby watch you while lying on a blanket just in front. She will delight at the sight of you in this very playful-looking position!

**Cesarean Variation:** You can start to assume this position at 4 weeks post-op. Wait until 8 weeks post-op to start the leg lifts, however, to avoid unnecessary strain on the forming scar.

*Note: If you have wrist pain or a history of carpal tunnel syndrome, fold back your yoga mat or place a folded towel under the heel of your hands so that the fingers are hanging off, to reduce the angle of wrist extension.

# The Plank

*This static position works nearly every muscle in the body simultaneously with almost no impact.*

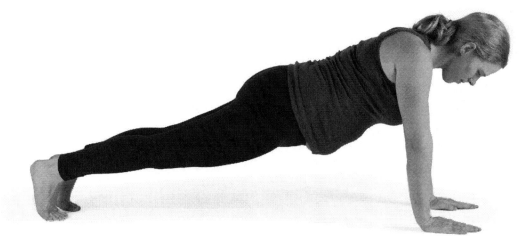

**Position:** From hands and knees, step one foot back followed by the other to stand on the balls of the feet with knees straight. Bring your hips down into line with the rest of your body to the "push-up" position. There should be a straight line from your shoulders to your hips to your knees to your ankles. Your hands should be directly under the shoulders.

**Action:** Just holding this position is exercise in itself. Focus on pushing up with the backs of the knees and reaching back with both heels. Draw the belly button in toward the spine and look at a point just forward of your hands to keep the neck relaxed. Breathe deeply and continuously. Hold this position for 5 breaths. Start with 3 reps, work up to 5. If the weight bearing hurts your wrists, try doing a rep or two up on your fists. The hands and wrists will usually get used to the weight bearing in just a few sessions. If you have carpal tunnel syndrome, practice the Plank on your fists, or modify the position by placing a folded hand towel under the heels of the hands to reduce the angle of wrist extension. If you are, or become, as your pregnancy progresses, unable to hold the body in a straight line, practice a modified Plank by dropping to your knees and lifting your feet as pictured below, always keeping a straight line in your body from the shoulders through the hips to the knees. Trembling is good.

**Using Your Baby Weight:** Position your baby on a folded towel or blanket under face, so you can look right at her while holding the pose. She will thoroughly enjoy your undivided attention. If you place her on her tummy facing you, she will have the motivation to lift her head and extend her trunk to watch you.

**Progression:** When you can comfortably perform 5 reps of Plank for 5 breaths you can try Plank with Leg Lifts (pg. 150).

**Cesarean Variation:** Due to the strong nature of the core contraction, wait until 6 weeks post op to perform the modified version of the Plank on your knees (fig. 2). Progress to the full Plank only when you are able to maintain the strong straight line in the body in the modified position for 5 breaths and 5 reps without discomfort in the incision, not before 8 weeks post-op.

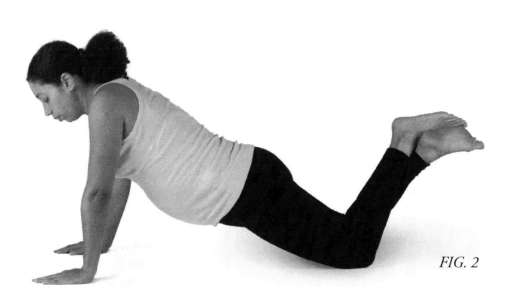

*FIG. 2*

# Lunge Flow

*This series of exercises strengthens and stretches most major muscle groups in the hips and legs. Work it in between the Quadruped and Plank position exercises. Variety is the key to combatting muscle soreness and boredom!*

**Position:** From hands and knees position, walk your hands over to the right side a few inches to make space to step your left foot forward beside your hands. Hands are positioned directly under the shoulders.

1. Drop your pelvis forward and walk hands forward if necessary to allow the front of the right hip to move toward the floor. Breathe 5 deep breaths, allowing the hip to sink deeper as you exhale. Move your hands up to the knee if it helps you to enjoy this hip stretch (fig. 1).
2. On the next inhalation, tuck the right toes under and press through the hands and right foot to lift the right knee (fig. 2). Activate the entire right leg by pressing up toward the ceiling with the back of the knee and reaching back with the heel. Focus on a point just out in front of you. Breathe 5 more deep breaths in this position. If your wrists hurt with the weight bearing, try this up on your fists.
3. Lower the right knee slowly back to the ground.
4. Relax the foot and walk your hands back toward you to straighten the left knee as you sit back toward your right heel (fig. 3). Release your head and neck, so that the forehead falls forward between the outstretched arms. You should feel a strong but tolerable stretch in the hamstring muscles on the back of the left thigh. Breathe 5 more deep breaths there, keeping the left knee straight.
5. Inhale as you lift your chest and walk the hands forward, releasing the front of the right hip forward and down toward the ground again (fig. 1) for 5 more breaths. Add an Elevator Kegel contraction for the 5 breaths. Repeat the rest of the series. Start with just these 2 reps on each side and work your way up to 5. You can mix these reps in with other exercises in Quadruped or Plank positions, but do at least 2 in a row on one side to get true lengthening of the muscles.

**Using Your Baby Weight:** Position your baby on a folded towel or blanket just in front of you. She'll enjoy some tummy time, developing head and neck control as she strengthens her neck and back extensors while watching you flow through this series.

**Cesarean Variation:** Begin only the hamstring stretch (fig. 3) portion of this series at 4 weeks post-op, until 6 weeks post-op when you can attempt the full flow as long as you don't have discomfort in the incision.

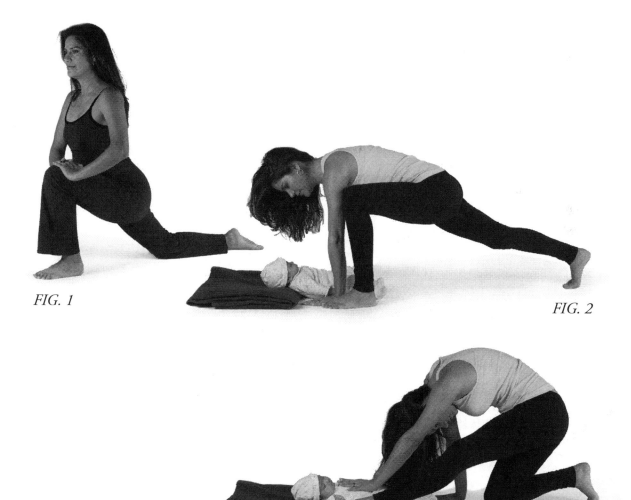

FIG. 1

FIG. 2

FIG. 3

# Plank with Leg Lift

*This variation of the Plank kicks it up a notch for the core requirements.*

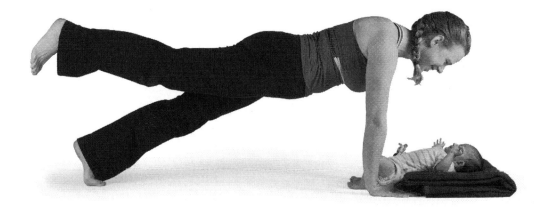

**Position:** Plank position (as described on pg. 146).

**Action:** Inhale as you shift your weight to one foot and exhale to slowly lift the other foot just a few inches off the floor. Inhale to lower the leg and shift your weight to the opposite side, exhale to lift the other leg. Repeat, alternating, for 3 reps in the beginning, working your way up to 10 on each side. After you can do the full 10 reps, try holding the leg up for a full breath each time, then two breaths, for fewer reps. Remember, trembling is good!

**Using Your Baby Weight:** Position your baby on a folded towel or blanket under your upper body, so that her face is just forward of yours when in position. Use this time to strike up a conversation with your infant. Talking helps avoid the tendency to hold your breath, and allows you and your infant to share a delightful interaction.

**Cesarean Variation:** Start with the modified Plank position at 6 weeks post-op and proceed first to Plank, then to the Plank with Leg Lift when you can do 5 reps for 5 breaths in the full Plank position without discomfort, not before 8 weeks post-op.

# Modified Push Ups

*A challenge for the core muscles and the upper body.*

**Position:** Modified Plank Position: On hands and knees with hips in line with the body, hands directly under shoulders, feet up. Get there from hands and knees by walking the hands forward about 6 inches then dropping the hips forward and down toward the floor to make a straight line from the shoulders through the hips to the knees. Or from Plank, simply drop the knees and lift the feet, crossing the ankles if you wish.
**Action:** Once in position, inhale deeply. Exhale as you bend the elbows, lowering your

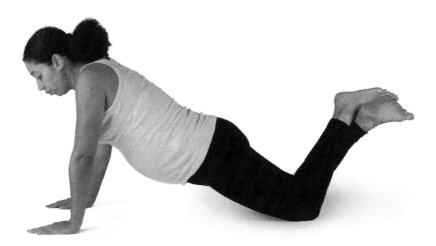

face toward the floor, keeping the elbows in close to the body. Only go as low as you can maintain the straight line in the body. Inhale to push yourself back up, keeping the straight line from shoulders to hips to knees as you rise. Repeat, using the whole exhalation to lower down and the whole inhalation to rise.

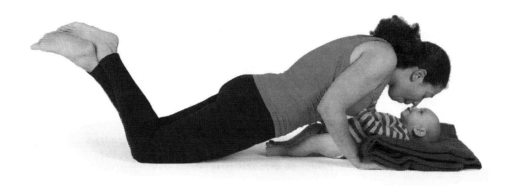

**Progression:** Start with only 3 reps, working your way up to 5 reps for as many as 4 or 5 sets during a session, not consecutive but interspersed with other exercises.

**Postpartum Progression:** After you can comfortably do 3 sets of 5 reps scattered through your routine, try to do Full Push Ups (pg.157).

**Using Your Baby Weight:** Position your baby on a folded towel or blanket under your upper body, so that her face is just forward of yours when in position. She will love it if you kiss her as you lower down.

**Cesarean Variation:** Try the static Modified Plank position without doing the push up starting at 6 weeks post-op if you have no pain at the incision site, to prepare your body for the Plank. Start the Modified Push Ups when you can hold the Modified Plank for 5 breaths and 5 reps.

**advanced – postpartum only**

*Add the following exercises only after you can do 5 reps of Plank for 5 breaths as well as Plank with Leg Lifts and Modified Push Ups for 5 reps without difficulty.*

**Using your Baby Weight:** Your baby can be on her belly or her back on a blanket just in front of you for this series. She will love this face-to-face interaction.

**Cesarean Variation:** Wait until 8 weeks post-op, and only after you can do Plank, Modified Push Ups, and Plank with Leg Lifts for 5 reps each without discomfort at the incision site.

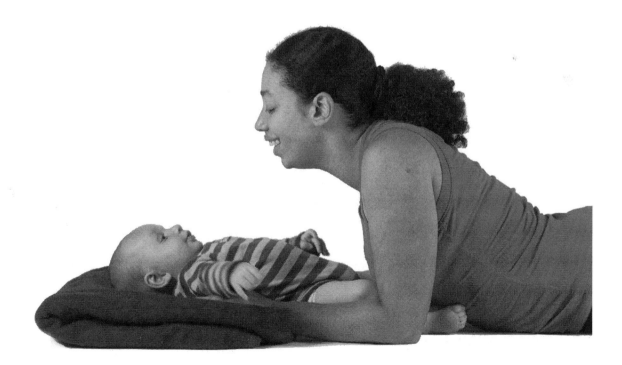

# Plank on Elbows

*Isolating the core in a no-impact highly effective pose.*

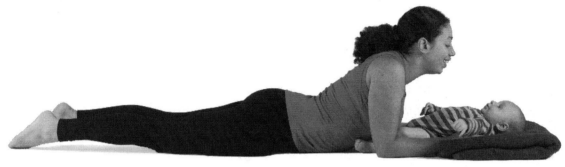

*FIG. 1*

**Position:** Lying face down, propped with your elbows under the shoulders, forearms parallel, palms down.

**Action:** First enjoy the relaxing position (fig.1) for a breath or two, allowing the chest to open forward as the shoulder blades come together toward the spine. As you exhale, tuck your toes under and lift the hips to the Plank position (fig. 2), stepping the feet in as needed to make a straight line in the body from the shoulders through the hips, through the knees and ankles, out the bottom of the heels. Visually focus on your baby slightly ahead of you on the floor. Mentally focus on maintaining calm and continuous deep breaths. Stay in the position for 5 deep breaths before lowering the hips to rest. Remember, trembling is good!

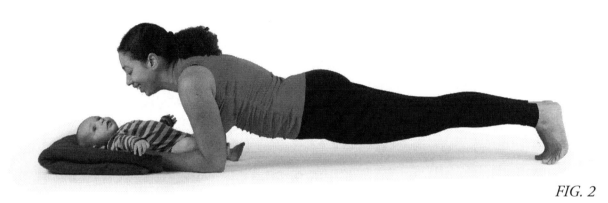

*FIG. 2*

**Progression:** Repeat for 3 reps, working your way up to 5 reps of 5 breaths. When you can comfortably do 5 reps of 5 breaths, try Leg Lifts in Plank on Elbows.

# Leg Lifts in Plank on Elbows

*Add this exercise when you can do 5 reps of Plank on Elbows for 5 breaths.*

**Position:** Plank on Elbows (pg. 154)

**Action:** After a deep breath in Plank on Elbows, inhale deeply to shift weight to one foot. Exhale to lift the opposite foot just 10 – 12 inches off the floor, keeping the knee straight. Lower the leg as you inhale and shift the weight to the opposite foot; exhale as you lift the other leg. Alternate the leg lifts with your breath, lifting as you exhale, lowering and shifting as you inhale, for 2-3 reps on each side at first. Work your way up to 5 reps each side. Keep the hips in line with the body throughout the exercise.

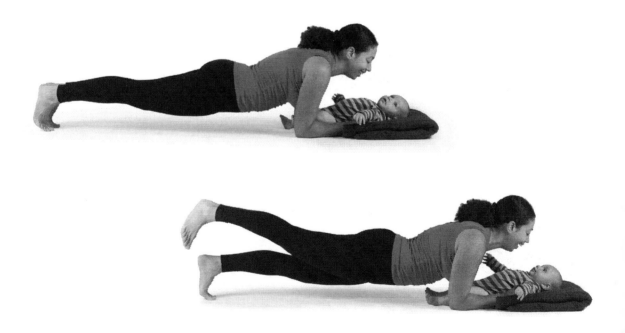

# Full Push Ups

*Add this exercise when you can easily do 5 reps of Modified Push Ups and 5 reps of The Plank for 5 breaths.*

**Position:** Plank position (pg. 146)

**Action:** Keep your elbows close to your body as you exhale to bend your elbows and lower your face toward the floor, only lowering as far as you can maintain the straight line in the body from the shoulders to the heels. Inhale, focusing on activating the abdominal muscles, drawing the navel in toward the spine to keep a strong straight line in the body as you push yourself back up to Plank.

**Progression:** Start with 3 reps of a shallow Push Up, working up to 5 reps of a deeper Push Up. Eventually incorporate 5 sets of 5 reps scattered throughout your routine.

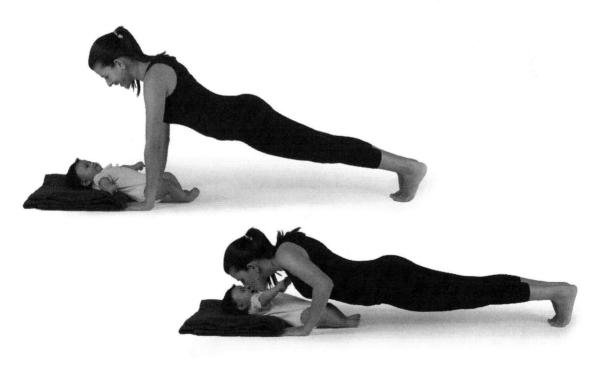

# Flying Pigeon Flow

*This dynamic series combines strong core work with a heavenly hip stretch.*

**Position:** Start in Downward Facing Dog (see pg. 144).

**Action:**

1. Breathe two deep breaths in Downward Facing Dog (fig. 1).
2. Inhale to lift the right leg, stacking the right hip directly on top of the left (fig. 2).
3. Exhale to bring the hips forward and down to more of a Plank position, moving the left foot back further as necessary, as you draw the right knee in toward the left elbow, taking care to keep the knee up high above your baby (fig. 3).
4. As you inhale, fly the leg back up behind you, stacking the hip as in fig. 2.
5. Exhale to repeat, bringing the hips forward and the knee toward the opposite elbow (fig. 3). Repeat in rhythm with the breath for 3 – 5 reps. On the last repetition, from the forward position (fig. 3) lower the right knee to the floor to the right of your baby and lower the hips so that they square off in the same plane with the floor, in the Pigeon pose (fig. 4). Stay there for at least 5 deep breaths. Repeat on the opposite side.

**Progression:** Start with 3 reps and work your way up to 8-10 on each side as you grow stronger. For added challenge, on the last rep before settling into the Pigeon pose, try holding the knee up as close as you can to the opposite elbow for a full breath, or two, or three! When you are able to hold the knee up on the last rep for 3 breaths, after one deep breath, try to pump the knee, lifting it higher off the ground as you forcefully exhale while in the forward position (fig. 3), starting with 3 pumps and working up to 10, for an intense oblique muscle challenge.

**Using Your Baby Weight:** Position your baby lying on her back or belly on a folded towel or blanket in front of you. She will enjoy the dynamic nature of this series and the look of determination on your face as you maintain the strong core contraction.

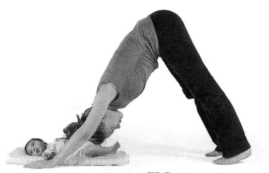

FIG. 1

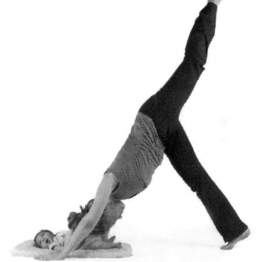

FIG. 2

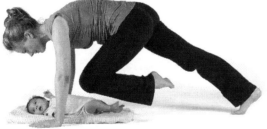

FIG. 3

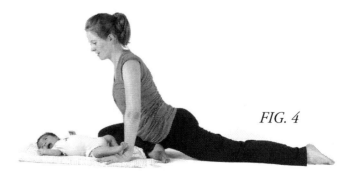

FIG. 4

# Standing Series

beginner level

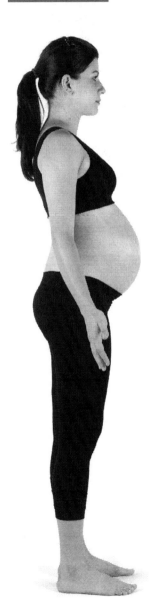

## Mountain Pose & Centering Breaths

*Correct your posture with this static yoga pose and practice the centering breaths to set your intention before proceeding with the dynamic standing exercises. Stand in the Mountain Pose throughout the day to align the spine and combat the common postural changes and resulting aches and pains of pregnancy.*

**Position:** Standing with feet hip-width apart, hands by sides.

**Action:** Inhale deeply as you tuck your tailbone under slightly and imagine a string pulling you from the crown of the head upward toward the sky, lengthening the spine. Exhale to roll your shoulders back and down, opening the heart, rotating the palms of the hands to face forward. Inhale your arms out to the sides and up overhead, imagining that you are gathering all the energy around you and bringing it together between your hands, allowing your gaze to follow your hands upward. Exhale as you join your hands and draw the energy with your hands into your heart. Repeat for 4 or 5 breaths, inhaling the arms out to the sides and up overhead, exhaling the hands to the heart. Add the Elevator Kegel to this exercise, drawing up and inward to take the elevator to the top as you exhale the hands to the heart, and hold it through several deep breaths.
**Using Your Baby Weight:** Leave your baby lying face up or

face down on a blanket, just in front of your feet. After several centering breaths, you can move from this pose into the next exercises, The Forward Bend and Row Baby, where you will actually *use* the baby's weight.

**Cesarean Note:** This exercise is safe to do as soon as day 3 after surgery without the arm movement and day 10 post-op with the arm movement, as long as you don't feel any uncomfortable pulling at the incision site. It is good to practice erect posture in the early days post-op so as not to make a habit of giving into the discomfort in the abdomen and developing poor posture and scar adhesions. If you feel discomfort with the arm movements, practice only deep breaths in the standing posture with the heart open and hands facing forward for a few more days.

# Pelvic Rocking

*Mobilizes the lumbar spine and pelvis, reversing the swayback curve and combating low back ache.*

**Position:** Standing with knees bent, hands on the thighs just above the knees.

**Action:** Inhale as you lift your chin and your sit bones, exaggerating the swayback curve (fig.1), then exhale as you rotate the sit bones downward to tuck your tailbone under (fig. 2). Avoid rounding the shoulders to focus the movement in the pelvis. Repeat for 8 to 10 breaths. After a few reps, add basic Kegel contractions, drawing in as you exhale and relaxing as you inhale.

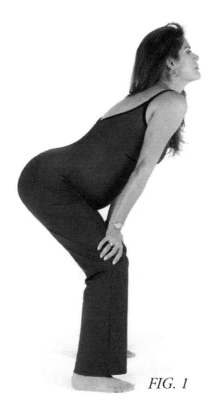

*FIG. 1*

**Using Your Baby Weight:** Because you need the support of both hands on the thighs to help isolate the movement to the pelvis, it is best to leave your baby on the floor on a folded blanket for this exercise and then move into the Forward Bend where you can lift her for added resistance (The Row Baby). However, you can do this exercise with your baby in a front carrier if you already have her there. Pelvic Rocking before and after walking for cardio exercise activates the abdominals and prevents low backache.

**Cesarean Variation:** It is safe to perform this exercise at 2 weeks post-op as long as you don't feel any uncomfortable pulling in the area of the incision.

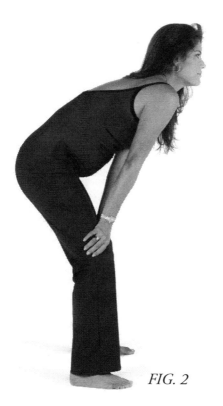

*FIG. 2*

# Forward Bend and Row Baby

*Stretches the low back and the backs of the thighs and strengthens postural muscles to help you stand up straight with less conscious effort.*

**Position:** Standing in Mountain Pose. If you have a big belly already, you may have to widen your stance to make room for it as you fold forward.

**Action:** Inhale the arms out to sides and up overhead. As you exhale, lead with the chest and open the arms out to the sides and back behind you, as if you are spreading your wings, and bend forward from the waist. Keep the knees slightly bent at first, then re-lease the hands toward the floor as if trying to touch your toes. Release the crown of the head toward the ground (fig. 1). Gently shake the head "yes" and "no" to help release all tension in the neck and shoulders. Breathe a few deep breaths in this position, gently taking the knees straight.

Inhale as you lift your heart up about halfway to make the spine straight, squeezing the shoulder blades together and lifting the head to look straight ahead (fig. 3). Exhale back down to touch the toes. Repeat, inhaling up to a flat back, exhaling down to try to touch the toes. Start with 3 – 5 reps. Work your way up to 10.

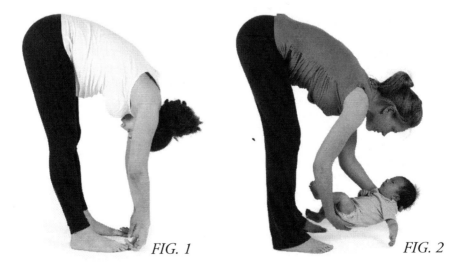

*FIG. 1*                                    *FIG. 2*

**Using Your Baby Weight – The Row Baby:** After performing 5 reps of the Forward Bend as described above, bend your knees deeply to allow you to reach down and pick up your baby, face down or face up (fig. 2). Draw the baby in close to your chest then take your knees almost straight, and lift up to the flat back position (fig. 4). Keep your back straight as you exhale slowly and straighten the arms to lower the baby back down toward the floor (fig. 3). Inhale to draw the baby in toward the chest again (fig. 4), exhale to lower the baby down (fig. 3), and repeat for 5 reps with the breath. Draw your belly button in toward your spine to protect your low back in this position.

**Cesarean Variation:** You will likely not feel comfortable in this position of extreme forward flexion for the first 3 – 4 weeks post-op. Do not add the baby weight until at least 6 weeks postpartum.

**\*Note:** If you feel lightheaded during this exercise, sit on the floor or stand while holding onto something for balance until the dizziness passes. If you have low blood pressure, skip this exercise until your blood pressure is within normal limits.

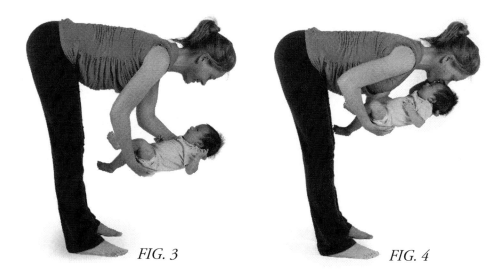

*FIG. 3*                                    *FIG. 4*

# Full Squats

*This hip opener is the most effective way to increase the size of the pelvic outlet to prepare for giving birth, and the best position to strengthen the pelvic floor muscles against gravity. Use positioning aids as needed to make yourself comfortable in this position, as the key to its success is staying for several deep breaths and practicing it often.*

**Position:** Start standing with feet wider than the hips, toes pointed out on a diagonal.

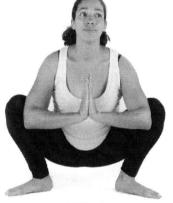

*FIG. 1*

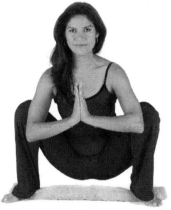

*FIG. 2*

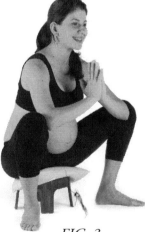

*FIG. 3*

**Action:** Gently bend the knees and lower the pelvis toward the floor, allowing your weight to fall back onto the heels. Bring the hands together in front of the chest, with the elbows in front of the knees gently pressing the knees open (fig. 1). Imagine a string pulling you from the crown of your head up toward the ceiling, your spine growing longer. If you can't get your heels down flat, place a towel roll under the heels (fig. 2). If you find you can't go down far enough on your own or have a hard time balancing, practice squatting with your rear supported on a small stool (fig. 3), or try regular squats while holding on to a table or other stable support. Stay in the pose for several deep breaths, at least 5 to start, gradually increasing to 30 breaths. Practice all variations of the Kegel exercises in this position.

**\*Note:** Avoid this position altogether if you have any complications such as full or partial placenta previa, vulvitis, active hemorrhoids, or a cervical suture. It is also best to avoid it during the last few weeks of pregnancy if your cervix has already started to dilate, to avoid inducing labor. Some health care practitioners recommend to practice only supported squats on a stool for the last 4-6 weeks of pregnancy to reduce pressure on the cervix and the pelvic floor. However, if you have reached your due date and want to encourage baby to come, spending time in Full Squats can help.

**Postpartum Progression:** This exercise is not indicated in the first weeks or even months postpartum. After giving birth, the last thing you want is to open the pelvic outlet, as many women often complain of feeling like their bottom is falling out. Just skip this one altogether until about 4 months postpartum and keep practicing your Kegel exercises to rehabilitate the pelvic floor. If by 4 months postpartum you are able to isolate the Kegel contractions and perform the variations of basic Kegel contractions as well as the Elevator, you will be ready to resume squatting and can progress your pelvic floor muscle training to include Kegel exercises in the squatting position at that time. If you experience pain in the pubic symphysis when first resuming the full squat, wait for another week or so and try again.

# Wide Leg Squats

*Builds strong legs and realigns the spine for better posture*

**Position:** Standing with legs much wider than your hips, toes pointed out at a 45 degree angle, hands reaching up toward the corners of the room as in fig. 1.

**Action:** Inhale deeply through the nose, gently tucking the tailbone under for a slight pelvic tilt. Exhale, bending the knees deeply to squat down as far as you can comfortably, making soft fists with the hands as you bend the elbows and squeeze the shoulder blades together (fig. 2). Inhale to push yourself back to standing as you reach up and out with the hands (fig. 1). Incorporate Kegel contractions, drawing in and upward from the perineum as you exhale to squat, and release as you inhale to stand.

**Using Your Baby Weight:** Gently cradle your small infant in your arms as you perform the squats (fig. 3), or support her in a front carrier and incorporate this exercise into a walking routine. After you can do 10 reps holding your baby, try the Chest Press, pressing her away from your chest as you exhale to squat (fig. 4), and pulling her close to your chest as you inhale to stand, supporting her head as needed.

**Cesarean Variation:** Wait until 3 weeks post op to start this exercise and do it *without* holding the baby for the first week. Avoid the Chest Press until 6 weeks post op.

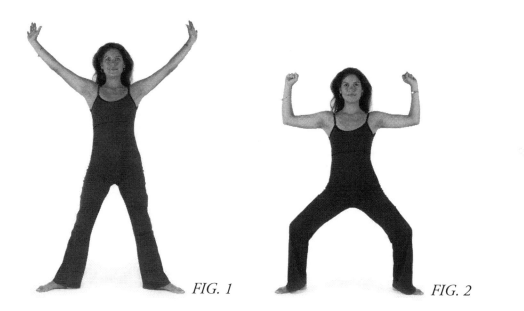

FIG. 1

FIG. 2

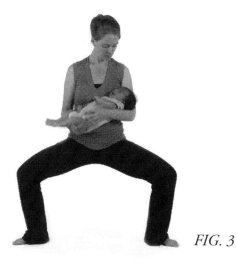

FIG. 3

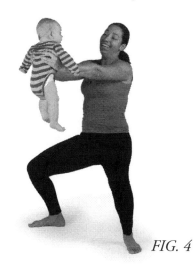

FIG. 4

# The Chair

*Feel the burn of this quadriceps contraction, for firmer thighs and a straighter spine.*

**Position:** Start standing with feet hip width apart, palms at sides.

**Action:** Inhale to lift both hands, reaching up and forward (when not holding your baby). Exhale to weight your seat and bend your knees, moving your sit bones downward toward the ground as if you are going to sit in a chair (fig. 1). Lift the toes at first to help shift the weight into the heels. Stay in the position for several deep breaths, moving deeper into the pose as you feel stronger and more confident. Try to keep your back straight and your weight in your heels. Remember, trembling is good! Incorporate Kegel exercises into this strong pose for pelvic floor toning. After one full breath in the pose, practice The Elevator Kegel contraction for several breaths.

**Progression:** Start with 5 breaths and 3 repetitions, gradually increasing reps and breaths to 10. If you find this exercise too difficult in the beginning, try the Cesarean variation described below for the first week or so to build strength and endurance in the muscles.

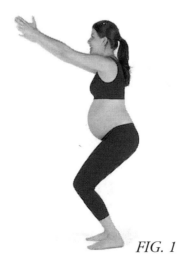

*FIG. 1*

**Using Your Baby Weight:** Cradle your baby in your arms while sitting back into The Chair pose (fig. 2). Start this variation only after you can perform 10 reps without holding the baby. When you feel stronger, try holding your baby under her arms out in front of you at shoulder height (fig. 3). You will have to decrease the number of breaths you hold the pose when you start this variation. Later still, you can start Chest Presses, pushing the baby out as you exhale and pulling her back into your chest as you inhale while holding the pose.

**Cesarean Variation:** You can begin a modified version of this exercise at 3 weeks post-op. Stand with your back flat against a wall and step your feet out about a foot and half to the front. Slide your back down the wall as you bend your knees, pressing your back flat into the wall. Don't let your knees go forward past your toes. Hold the position for 5 deep breaths before pushing through the feet to slide the back up the wall to stand. Repeat 3 – 5 times to start, working gradually up to 10 breaths and 10 reps.

You can begin the exercise away from the wall at 4 weeks post op, without holding your baby, as long as you don't experience any uncomfortable pulling in the scar. Add the resistance of the baby weight after 6 weeks post op, only when you can comfortably perform 10 reps for 5 breaths.

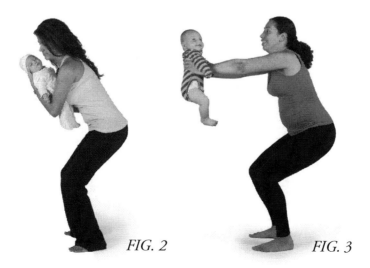

*FIG. 2*          *FIG. 3*

# Sciatic Stretch

*As the name implies, this stretch mobilizes the sciatic nerve all along its path from the lumbosacral spine down the back of the leg to provide relief from and to prevent sciatic pain.*

**Position:** Standing with the feet crossed and the knees as straight as they can be, trying to bring the toes of both feet in line with one another.

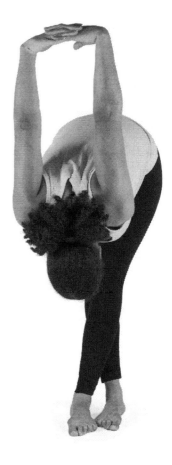

**Action:** Take hands behind the back and interlace the fingers. Inhale deeply while you roll the shoulders back to open the chest. Exhale as you fold forward at the waist, releasing the crown of the head toward the floor. Inhale again to lift the hands up behind you for a strong shoulder stretch. Stay in this position for 3 – 5 breaths. Lower the hands to rest on the sacrum if the stretch becomes uncomfortable in the shoulders. Release the hands before slowly rising to stand. Repeat with the opposite leg in front, for 3 to 5 reps on each side.

**\*Note:** During pregnancy, you will find it increasingly difficult to achieve a stretch in this position as your belly grows. When you no longer feel comfortable in this position, discontinue this stretch until after baby comes and do instead the Piriformis Stretch described on pg. 173.

**Using Your Baby Weight:** Position your baby on a folded towel or blanket in front of your feet for this stretch.

**Cesarean Note:** It is safe to perform this stretch once it feels comfortable, after your stitches are removed. It will usually be 2 to 3 weeks before this will feel good. Don't rush it. You have plenty of time. If you are experiencing sciatic pain and this position is uncomfortable, try instead the Legs up the Wall (pg. 82) and the Piriformis Stretch (pg. 173).

# Chapter 7: Soothing Mommy's Woes: Remedies for Common Aches, Pains, and Maladies

## Sciatica

Many women experience sciatic nerve pain during and after pregnancy due changes in pelvic shape and position and muscle tightness in the deep hip rotators. The pain is a deep ache often felt in one buttock, sometimes radiating down the back of the leg to the calf or all the way to the heel.

**Remedy:** Stretch the deep hip rotator muscles at least twice a day for 30 seconds and 3 reps each. Try the Sciatic Stretch as described on pg. 172. Another option is the Piriformis Stretch: Place a towel or belt around the back of the right thigh. Place the left ankle on the right knee and use the towel or belt to pull the right knee in toward your chest. You may be able to do without the towel, using the hands behind the right thigh to pull the knee in toward the chest. You should feel a deep stretch in the left hip. Hold for 10 deep breaths, for 3 reps on each side. You can also try this same stretch while sitting with the left ankle on the right knee, first sitting tall then gently leaning forward to feel a stretch deep in the left hip. If you feel any knee pain, stop.

## Round Ligament Spasm

Many pregnant women experience pain resulting from strain on the ligaments that anchor the uterus to the pelvis. It might feel like an ache or a sharp and shooting pain on one side, very low in the abdomen near the pubis, or in the groin. Round ligament pain often occurs with walking or exercise and with changing positions in the bed.

**Remedy:** The pain will usually subside with a few minutes rest. If recurring round ligament pain is affecting your ability to walk distances or to exercise, try an elastic support under your belly to reduce the strain on the ligaments. In bed, position yourself with a pillow under your belly for support, and take care to roll your body as a unit, the log roll maneuver, so that the hips and shoulders always move together to avoid twisting.

## Pubic Symphysis Pain

Later in pregnancy and after delivery, it is common to feel a pain in the joint where the two sides of the pelvis come together in the front at the pubis (see fig. 3 pg. 48), called the pubic symphysis. Misalignment of the pelvis is the most common cause of pain in that region. Pain is usually felt in the center where the bones join, but may also be felt in the groin on one or both sides, or in the sacroiliac joints where the sacrum meets the pelvis at the base of the spine.

**Remedy:** Avoid asymmetrical activities where the pelvis is oriented in opposite directions, as in some standing yoga poses. You can often realign the pelvis with a strong muscular contraction. Start with a Hug Your Knees Stretch (pg. 84) held for 10 counts, followed by Bridging (pg. 106) held for 10 counts, then place a pillow between your knees and squeeze your knees together, holding for 10 counts. Repeat up to 5 times twice a day. The Piriformis Stretch (pg. 173) and Hamstring Stretch (pg. 183) also help since they stretch muscles that also attach to the pelvis. If symptoms persist, seek treatment from a physical therapist to realign the pelvis with muscle energy techniques.

## Neck and Shoulder Pain and Tension

Postural changes during pregnancy and the physical demands of carrying a baby around cause an uncomfortable tightening of the muscles in the neck and shoulders. Some women have neck pain that can result in headaches. Others feel like their shoulders are drawn close to their ears, or have pain and tension between the shoulder blades.

**Remedy:** Practice the relaxation techniques outlined on pg. 79 – 82 at least once a day to help release mental and physical tension. The Neck and Shoulder stretches on page 123-124, practiced once or twice a day will help to lengthen tight muscles. Try to be conscious of your posture; avoid slouching. Strengthening exercises for the postural muscles can improve posture and reduce pain. Try the arm exercises listed on pg. 180 in the Bed Rest Program, as well as the Thread the Needle exercise on pg. 140 and Wide Legs Squats with the arm movement on pg. 168 – 169.

## Low Back Pain

The shift in the body's center of gravity, tightening of the lumbar musculature, and overstretching of the abdominal muscles predispose the pregnant woman to low back pain. The pain may manifest as an achy tightness in the lumbar muscles or a sharper pain in one or both of the sacroiliac joints (the place where the base of the spine meets the pelvis, often marked by dimples).

**Remedy:** Do at least 3 of the following stretches twice a day for 30 seconds and 3 reps each: Legs up the Wall (pg. 82), Wide Leg and Side Leg Stretches (pg. 121 – 122), Hug Your Knees and Happy Baby Stretches (pg. 84 – 85), and the Piriformis Stretch (pg. 173). Strengthen the abdominal muscles with the CoreMama™ exercises. Be sure to use good body mechanics: Bend your knees to lift, kneel or squat to do low activities, and try to hold your baby close to your body in front, not to one side. Use a front carrier even around the house to avoid unnecessary strain.

## Stress Incontinence

Overstretching of the pelvic floor muscles and pressure from the uterus on the bladder can cause bladder incontinence during pregnancy that may persist afterward due to pelvic floor weakness. Many women experience urinary leakage, especially when the intra-abdominal pressure increases with a cough or sneeze.

**Remedy:** Kegel exercises can help to maintain and recover pelvic floor muscle tone. See pg. 51 for a detailed description of the different types of Kegel contractions. Practice at least 100 a day, every day. If you have difficulty with the Kegel exercises or feel you have a more serious pelvic floor disorder, seek treatment from a physical therapist specializing in women's health issues to help you to isolate and strengthen the pelvic floor musculature.

## Swollen, Achy Feet and Ankles

Fluid retention and decreased venous circulation make swelling in the lower extremities common, especially during the late stages of pregnancy and in warmer climates. Lax ligaments can cause flattening of the arches and achiness in the feet.

**Remedy:** Get off your feet frequently throughout the day. Practice Legs Up the Wall (pg. 82) several times a day, and Ankle Pumps, Circles and the Alphabet (pg. 178). Mobilize the toes, help restore the arches, and increase circulation by placing a towel on the floor under your foot while sitting, and practice pulling the towel back with your toes to scrunch the towel.

## Leg Cramps

Aching pains and sharp, seizing cramps in the backs of the thighs and calf muscles are common especially in the last trimester of pregnancy.

**Remedy:** Take supplements of potassium, calcium, and magnesium. Stretch your calf muscles daily by standing facing a wall with one foot forward, the back heel down and toes facing forward, hands on the wall. Lean into the wall to stretch the back leg. Hold for 10 breaths. Repeat 3 times on each side. Legs up the Wall with Ankle Pumps (pg. 82) can also help by increasing circulation.

## Sleep Disorders

Many women develop difficulty sleeping in the late stages of pregnancy due to aches, pains and general discomfort related to their expanding form.

**Remedy:** Try a change of position. Since it is not recommended to lie flat on your back after the first trimester for more than a few minutes, lying on your side with pillows for support is a good alternative for relaxation as well as for sleeping during pregnancy and afterward. Get comfortable on your side with a thick pillow between the knees to ease pressure on your low back and another pillow of appropriate thickness under the pregnant belly to support the weight of the baby. Try hugging a large pillow in front of you to release tension in the shoulders. One pillow under the head is probably enough to maintain a neutral position of the neck, so the head is not higher or lower than the line of the spine. Yet another pillow between the ankles might be in order, especially if you have had hip or sciatic pain. Once you are finally in position with all pillows in place, close your eyes and turn your focus inward to the breath. You might be sleeping before the third breath, the relaxation effect is so profound. This is also an excellent position for laboring, according to the Bradley Method of natural childbirth[19] as the relaxation of all skeletal muscles allows the body to advance more rapidly in the active phase of labor.

# Chapter 8: The Alternative to Rest: Exercises for Women on Bed Rest

You might be placed on bed rest restrictions for a variety of medical reasons at some point during your pregnancy. While this restriction can drastically limit your mobility, it doesn't mean that you can't exercise. There are several exercises you can safely perform while on bed rest that will help maintain joint range of motion and muscle tone and flexibility. The exercises give you something to do in a variety of positions, providing a welcome purpose for at least a few minutes of the day. Focusing on what you *can* do is good for your mental health as well.

If you have access to a physical therapist, she can provide you with individual instruction in safe mobility practices and can construct a personalized exercise program. If not, you can follow the exercises outlined below up to 3 times per day. You should always check with your prenatal health care provider before implementing any exercise program. Since there are many reasons for prescribing bed rest, every case is distinct and only your health practitioner can tell you which exercises are right for you. Show your health care provider the *Baby Weight* Bed Rest Program to determine specifically what you *are* allowed to do. Tune into BabyWeightTV™ to find classes based on this program for mamas on bed rest who have been cleared by their doctors to follow these gentle but effective exercises, at www.babyweight.tv.

## Kegel Exercises

Review the different types of Kegel exercises on pg.51. All are safe to perform while on bed rest in a variety of positions. Try to do a total of at least 200 a day to maintain good muscle tone and strength in the pelvic floor musculature.

# Supine Series

## Ankle Pumps/Ankle Alphabet

Helps keep ankles flexible and promotes lower extremity circulation. Lying on your back with legs straight, practice forcefully pumping the feet up and down, then in circles in both directions for 20 reps each. Afterwards pretend there is paint on your big toe and try to draw the alphabet one letter at a time by moving the feet.

## Shoulder Shrugs and Neck Mobility

To relieve neck and shoulder pain and release tension, do this exercise throughout the day.

1. Lift your shoulders up toward your ears as you inhale, then press them down toward your hips as you exhale. Repeat 20 times.
2. Exhale to turn your head to one side to try to line up the chin with the shoulder, then inhale the head back to the center. Exhale to the opposite side. Repeat 20 times.
3. Exhale to bend your neck to the side, dropping your ear toward your shoulder. Inhale back up to the center. Exhale to the opposite side. Repeat for 20 reps on each side.

## Pelvic Tilts

This exercise helps to maintain abdominal tone and pelvic mobility without increasing pressure on the uterus or cervix. Lying on your back with knees bent, press the low back flat. Hold for 10 counts. Repeat for 20 reps. Add Elevator Kegel contractions as you press the low back flat, and hold through the 10 counts before releasing (see pg. 88).

## Activate Transverse Abdominus

Lying on your back with the knees bent and the arms crossed over your belly so you can feel the space between the ribs and the pelvis, inhale deeply to inflate the abdomen. Exhale slowly and make an "ahhh" sound as you tighten the sides of the abdominal corset. You should feel the tightening in the waistband under your fingertips. Inhale to release the contraction. Repeat 20 times. See pg. 86 for a more detailed description.

## Short Arc Quads

Place a rolled pillow or blanket under your knees and alternate straightening one knee, then the other, to tighten the quadriceps muscle on the front of the thigh. Hold each contraction for 5 counts. Repeat 10-20 times each side.

## Straight Leg Raises

Lying on your back with one leg bent and one leg straight, propped in a semi-reclined position with 2 pillows under your head and upper back if it is more comfortable. Press the low back flat to activate a pelvic tilt, then lift the straight leg to the height of the opposite knee as you inhale. Hold for 3 counts before lowering slowly as you exhale. Repeat 10 – 20 reps on each side. Add Kegel contractions, drawing upward and inward in the perineum as you exhale and lower the leg, relaxing as you inhale and lift. You can add 1-pound ankle weights if 20 reps without weights is not difficult (see pg. 96).

## Heel Slides

Lying on your back with knees bent, press the low back flat then slowly slide one heel along the bed to make the knee straight as you exhale. Inhale to slide the heel along the bed toward your rear to bend the knee (see pg. 91). Repeat 10-20 reps on each side. Add Elevator Kegel contractions to hold through 5 to 10 breaths while doing Heel Slides. You can later add 1-pound ankle weights to increase muscle toning.

# Bridging

This exercise helps to keep your muscles strong for bed mobility and, when necessary, for using a bedpan. Lying on your back with knees bent, press through the feet to lift the hips as you exhale. Lower the hips slowly as you inhale. Integrate Kegel contractions, drawing in the perineum as you exhale to lift the hips, relaxing as you inhale to lower the hips. Repeat 10 – 20 reps. See pg. 106 for a detailed description.

# Legs Up the Wall

This is a good resting position, which stretches the legs and helps with lower extremity circulation. Lying on your back with your hips as close to the wall as they can be and the legs outstretched up the wall. Rest here for up to 10 minutes at a time, with a pillow under one hip to reduce pressure on the descending aorta if you want to stay in this position more than 3 minutes when you are more than 20 weeks pregnant. Practice Ankle Pumps and Circles in this position. See pg. 82 for a detailed description and variations.

# Arm Exercises

Lying on your back or propped in a semi-reclined position with 2 pillows under your head and upper back, with both knees bent.

1. Lift arms with elbows straight from your sides to up over your head as you inhale, lower them slowly as you exhale. Repeat for 20 reps.
2. Bring palms together with arms straight up over your chest. Inhale to open the arms and lower the hands out to the sides and down toward the bed. Exhale to bring the palms together up over your chest. Repeat for 20 reps.
3. With arms straight by the sides and palms facing upward, inhale to bend the elbows and bring the hands up toward the shoulders, exhale to lower the hands back down to the bed.Repeat for 20 reps.

*Add 1-pound weights to all of the arm exercises after you can do 20 reps without difficulty.

# SideLying Series

## Hip Abduction

Lying on your side with the top leg straight and the bottom leg bent, lift the top leg straight up to the side as you exhale, lower it slowly as you inhale. Add Kegel contractions, drawing inward in the perineum as you exhale and lift the leg, releasing as you inhale and lower the leg. Repeat 10 – 20 times. See pg. 131 for a detailed description.

## Hip Extension

Lying on your side with the bottom leg bent and the top leg straight and raised a few inches so it is at the level of the hip. Exhale to push the leg straight back behind you with the knee straight. Inhale the leg back in line with your body. Repeat 10 – 20 times.

## Hip Adduction

Lying on your side, propped on your elbow, with your top leg bent so that the top foot is placed flat in front of your thigh, using your hand at the ankle to stabilize the leg. Lock the bottom knee straight and lift the bottom leg up as you exhale. Lower the leg to the bed as you inhale. See pg. 133 for a detailed description. Add Kegel contractions, drawing inward in the perineum as you exhale and lift the leg, releasing as you inhale and lower the leg. Repeat for 10-20 reps.

*You can add 1-pound ankle weights to all leg exercises after performing 20 reps is no longer difficulty. You can easily make homemade weights. Cans of vegetables (14.oz) or bottles of water (16 – 20 oz) make great hand weights and weigh about a pound each. For the ankles, empty a pound of rice into a long sock or stocking and tie it off with a rubber band. Use a hair clip to fasten it around your ankle.

# Sitting Series

If you have bathroom privileges and are allowed to sit for at least a couple of minutes, take advantage by doing a few exercises while sitting.

## Leg Extension

While sitting on the edge of the bed, lift one foot to straighten the knee, tightening the thigh muscle. Hold for 3 counts before lowering slowly. Repeat for 10 – 20 reps. Add a 1-pound ankle weight for increased resistance if desired.

## Arm Exercises

You can do all of the Arm Exercises described on pg. 180 while sitting, as well as the following:

1. Place your hands on your shoulders and make backward circles with the elbows. Repeat for 20 reps.
2. Stretch your arms out to the sides at shoulder height and make large backward circles. Repeat for 20 reps.

## Shoulder and Neck Stretches

You can safely perform all of the Shoulder and Neck Stretches described on pg. 123 – 124 to relieve pain and muscular tension and to preserve posture while on bed rest. Hold each stretch for 5 breaths and repeat up to 5 times on each side.

1. Triceps Stretch: Reach up with the right hand then place it between the shoulder blades. Place the left hand on the right elbow and draw the elbow toward the left shoulder, behind the head.
2. Shoulder Rotator Stretch: Place the right hand between the shoulder blades from up above, and the left hand back behind you between the shoulder blades from down below. Try to touch and take hold of the fingertips of the opposite hand, or just take

hold of your shirt with each hand.

3.  Cervical Release: Drop your chin forward and rest one hand on the back of the head as you exhale. Don't pull. Breathe 5 deeps breaths then release the hand and inhale the head back up. Then drop the head to the right side as you exhale and rest the right hand on the left ear. Don't pull. Hold for 5 deeps breaths before releasing as you inhale. Repeat to the left side.

# Hamstring Stretch

Sit on the edge of the bed, with the right foot on the floor and the left leg outstretched on the bed. Flex the left foot back toward you and gently lean forward toward the left leg, reaching for your left foot. Hold for 5 deep breaths. Repeat 3-5 times on each side.

# References

[1] Rasmussen, K. M., Yaktine, A. L. (eds.), *Weight Gain During Pregnancy: Reexamining the Guidelines.* Washington, D.C.: National Academy Press, 2009.

[2] Hanula, G. M. "Building Baby's Brain: What to Eat When You're Expecting," The University of Georgia, Publication No. FACS 01-09, September 1998.

[3] American Heart Association. "Fish and Omega-3 Fatty Acids," Retrieved Jan. 28, 2010 from www.heart.org/HEARTORG/GettingHealthy/NutritionCenter/Healthy-DietGoals/Fish-and-Omega-3-Fatty-Acids_UCM_303248_Article.jsp

[4] Harvard School of Public Health, The Nutrition Source. "Fats and Cholesterol: Out with the Bad, In with the Good," Retrieved Jan. 20, 2010 from http://www.hsph.harvard.edu/nutritionsource/what-should-you-eat/fats-full-story/index.html

[5] Harvard School of Public Health, The Nutrition Source. "Fish, Friend or Foe?" Retrieved Jan. 20, 2010 from http://www.hsph.harvard.edu/nutritionsource/what-should-you-eat/fish/

[6] Harvard School of Public Health, The Nutrition Source. "Healthy Drinks," Retrieved Jan. 20, 2010 from http://www.hsph.harvard.edu/nutritionsource/healthy-drinks/

[7] Bodnar, J. "Sugar Substitutes During Pregnancy: Do Artificial Sweeteners and Pregnancy Mix?" *Pregnancy Today.* Retrieved March 18, 2011 from http://www.pregnancytoday.com/articles/pregnancy-nutrition-and-recipes/sugar-substitutes-during-pregnancy-3541/

[8] Agatston, A. S., *The South Beach Diet.* New York: Random House, 2003.

[9] Eiger, M.S., Olds, S. W., *The Complete Book of Breastfeeding,* 3rd ed., New York: Workman Publishing, 1999.

[10] March of Dimes. "Your Pregnant Body, Weight Gain During Pregnancy," Sept. 2009. Retreived July 28, 2010 from http://www.marchofdimes.com/pregnancy/your-body_weightgain.html

[11] Nygaard,I., Barber, M.D., Burgio, K.L., Kenton, K., Meikle, S., Schaffer, J., Spino, C., Whitehead, W.E., Wu, J., and Brody, D.J., "Prevalence of Symptomatic Pelvic Floor Disorders in U.S. Women," *Journal of the American Medical Asscociation,* Sept. 17 2008, Vol. 300, No. 11, Pages 1311-1316.

[12] Clapp, J.F., *Exercising Through Your Pregnancy.* Omaha: Addicus Books, 2002.

[13] The American Congress of Obstetricians and Gynecologists. "Exercise During Pregnancy and the Postpartum Period," ACOG Committee Opinion number 267, published Jan. 2002, reaffirmed 2009. Retrieved from http://mail.ny.acog.org/web-site/SMIPodcast/Exercise.pdf

[14] The American Congress of Obstetricians and Gynecologists. "Postpartum De-pression," ACOG Education Pamphlet AP091, January 2009. Retrieved June 2, 2010 from www.acog.org/publications/patient_education/bp091.cfm

[15] Wisner, K.L., Parry, B.L., and Piontek, C.M. "Postpartum Depression," *New England Journal of Medicine,* Vol. 347, No. 3, p. 194-199. July 18, 2002.

[16] Marcus, Sheila M. "Depression During Pregnancy: Rates, Risks and Conse-quences, Motherisk Update 2008," *Canadian Journal of Clinical Pharmacology,* Winter 2009, Vol.16, No.1, p. 15-22. Jan. 22, 2009.

[17] Armstrong K., Edwards H. "The Effectiveness of a Pram Walking Exercise Pro-gramme in Reducing Depressive Symptomology for Postnatal Women." *International Journal of Nursing Practice,* 2004; Vol. 10, No. 4, p. 177-194.

[18] Norman,E., Sherburn, M., Osborne, R.H., and Galea, M.P., "An Exercise and Education Program Improves Well-Being of New Mothers: A Randomized Controlled Trial," *Physical Therapy, Journal of the American Physical Therapy Association,* March 2010 Vol. 90 No. 3, p. 348-355.

[19] McCutcheon, S., *Natural Childbirth the Bradley Way,* revised ed., New York: Plume, 1996.

# Suggested Flows of CoreMama™ Exercises

You can find videos incorporating all the CoreMama™ exercises into fun and challenging classes for every skill level on BabyWeightTV™ at www.babyweight.tv. However, for more portability, you can use these suggested flows after you are familiar with the exercises. If you find an exercise too difficult or have any question or doubt about how to perform it correctly, refer back to the detailed description on the page numbers listed. Listen to your body and rest as often as needed between exercises. Use the modified positions described in the text as necessary. When the Plank position is pictured, for example, feel free to drop to your knees and do the Modified Plank instead if you find Plank too challenging. Only do the exercises that are within your ability. You can later add the more difficult exercises as you get stronger.

Some exercises are repeated in the flows to include more than one set in a session. The SideLying Series and Lunge Flow exercises, however, are meant to be done first on one side, then repeated later in the routine on the opposite side. All other bilateral exercises should done on both sides before proceeding to the next exercise in the flow.

Don't forget your pelvic floor! Remember to integrate the various types of Kegel exercises (pg. 51) into all the exercises demonstrated in the following suggested flows of the CoreMama™ exercises.

The diagrams on the following pages illustrate possible sequences of CoreMama™ Exercises. They should be read across both pages, from left-to-right, top-to-bottom:

**beginner level**

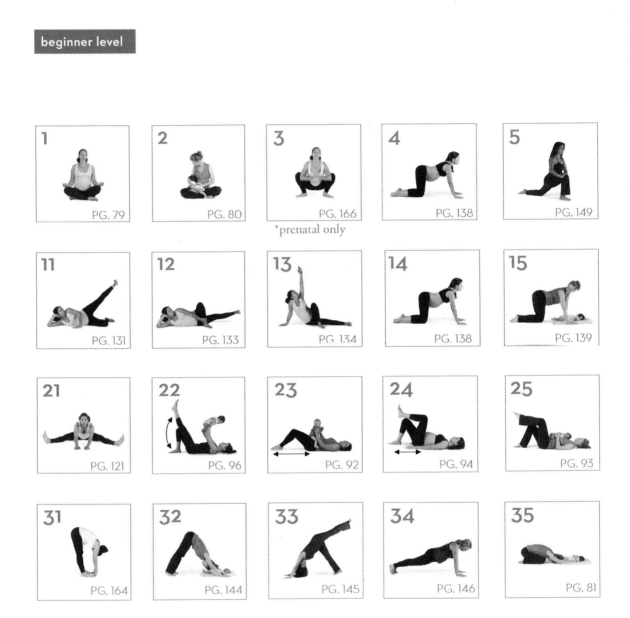

1    PG. 79

2    PG. 80

3    PG. 166
*prenatal only

4    PG. 138

5    PG. 149

11    PG. 131

12    PG. 133

13    PG. 134

14    PG. 138

15    PG. 139

21    PG. 121

22    PG. 96

23    PG. 92

24    PG. 94

25    PG. 93

31    PG. 164

32    PG. 144

33    PG. 145

34    PG. 146

35    PG. 81

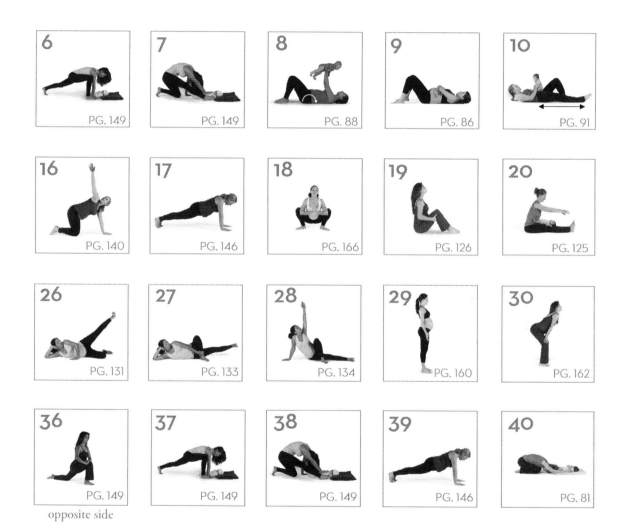

6   PG. 149

7   PG. 149

8   PG. 88

9   PG. 86

10   PG. 91

16   PG. 140

17   PG. 146

18   PG. 166

19   PG. 126

20   PG. 125

26   PG. 131

27   PG. 133

28   PG. 134

29   PG. 160

30   PG. 162

36   PG. 149

37   PG. 149

38   PG. 149

39   PG. 146

40   PG. 81

opposite side

**intermediate level**

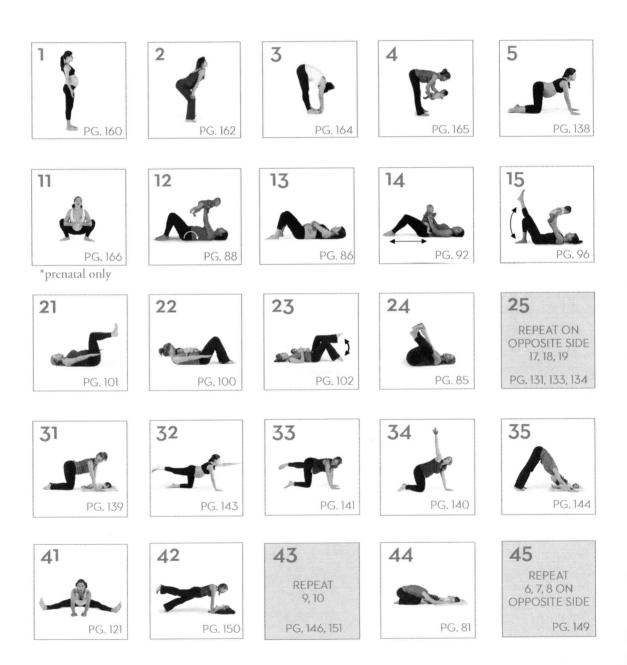

1 — PG. 160
2 — PG. 162
3 — PG. 164
4 — PG. 165
5 — PG. 138

11 — PG. 166
*prenatal only
12 — PG. 88
13 — PG. 86
14 — PG. 92
15 — PG. 96

21 — PG. 101
22 — PG. 100
23 — PG. 102
24 — PG. 85
25 — REPEAT ON OPPOSITE SIDE 17, 18, 19 — PG. 131, 133, 134

31 — PG. 139
32 — PG. 143
33 — PG. 141
34 — PG. 140
35 — PG. 144

41 — PG. 121
42 — PG. 150
43 — REPEAT 9, 10 — PG. 146, 151
44 — PG. 81
45 — REPEAT 6, 7, 8 ON OPPOSITE SIDE — PG. 149

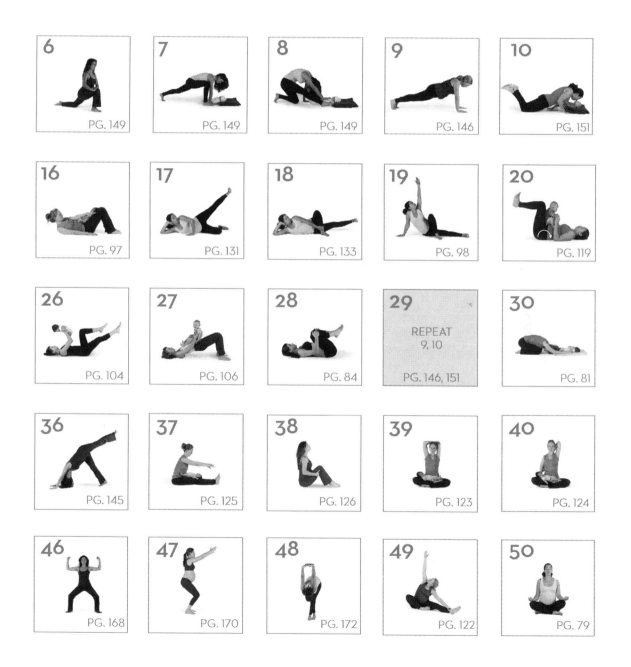

6    PG. 149

7    PG. 149

8    PG. 149

9    PG. 146

10    PG. 151

16    PG. 97

17    PG. 131

18    PG. 133

19    PG. 98

20    PG. 119

26    PG. 104

27    PG. 106

28    PG. 84

29    REPEAT 9, 10    PG. 146, 151

30    PG. 81

36    PG. 145

37    PG. 125

38    PG. 126

39    PG. 123

40    PG. 124

46    PG. 168

47    PG. 170

48    PG. 172

49    PG. 122

50    PG. 79

## advanced level

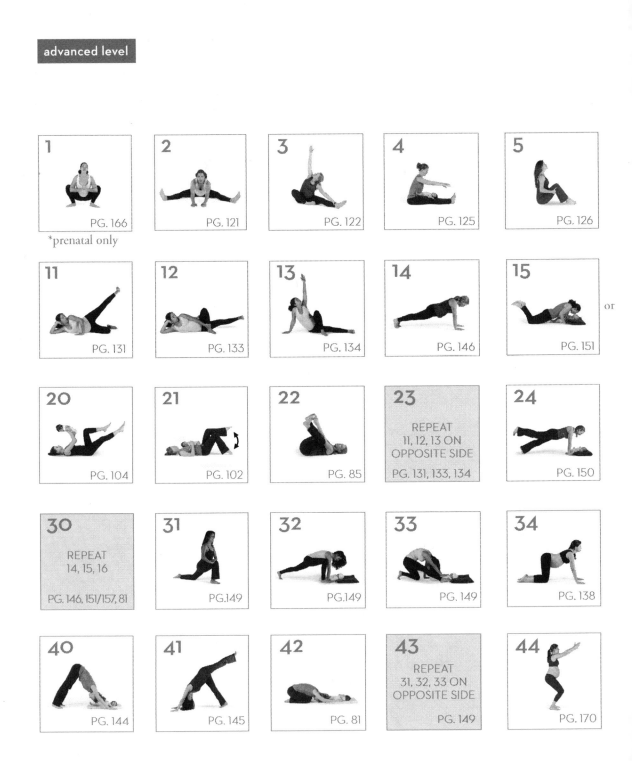

**1** PG. 166
*prenatal only

**2** PG. 121

**3** PG. 122

**4** PG. 125

**5** PG. 126

**11** PG. 131

**12** PG. 133

**13** PG. 134

**14** PG. 146

**15** PG. 151    or

**20** PG. 104

**21** PG. 102

**22** PG. 85

**23** REPEAT 11, 12, 13 ON OPPOSITE SIDE PG. 131, 133, 134

**24** PG. 150

**30** REPEAT 14, 15, 16 PG. 146, 151/157, 81

**31** PG. 149

**32** PG. 149

**33** PG. 149

**34** PG. 138

**40** PG. 144

**41** PG. 145

**42** PG. 81

**43** REPEAT 31, 32, 33 ON OPPOSITE SIDE PG. 149

**44** PG. 170

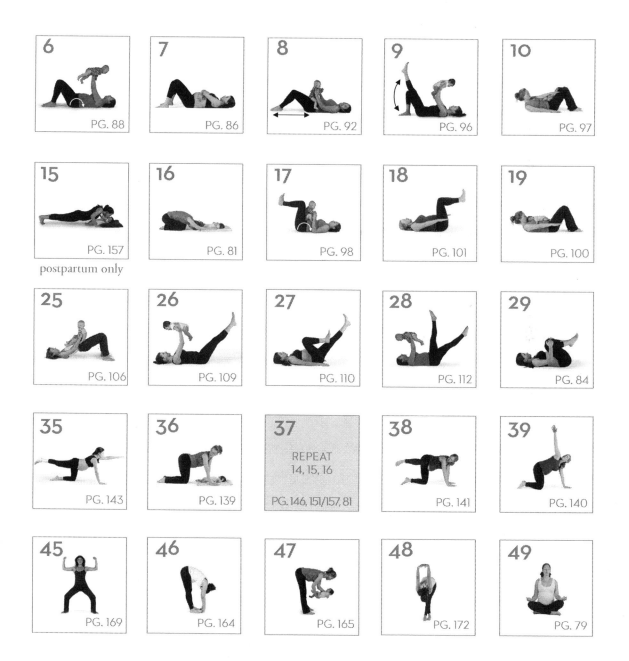

6    PG. 88
7    PG. 86
8    PG. 92
9    PG. 96
10   PG. 97

15   PG. 157
postpartum only
16   PG. 81
17   PG. 98
18   PG. 101
19   PG. 100

25   PG. 106
26   PG. 109
27   PG. 110
28   PG. 112
29   PG. 84

35   PG. 143
36   PG. 139
37   REPEAT 14, 15, 16   PG. 146, 151/157, 81
38   PG. 141
39   PG. 140

45   PG. 169
46   PG. 164
47   PG. 165
48   PG. 172
49   PG. 79

**postnatal only**

After you have had your baby and have worked up to the advanced level exercises, you can do the following exercises alone for a quick core-focused boost, but it's meant to be added to the previous Advanced Level flow for an intense postpartum work out.

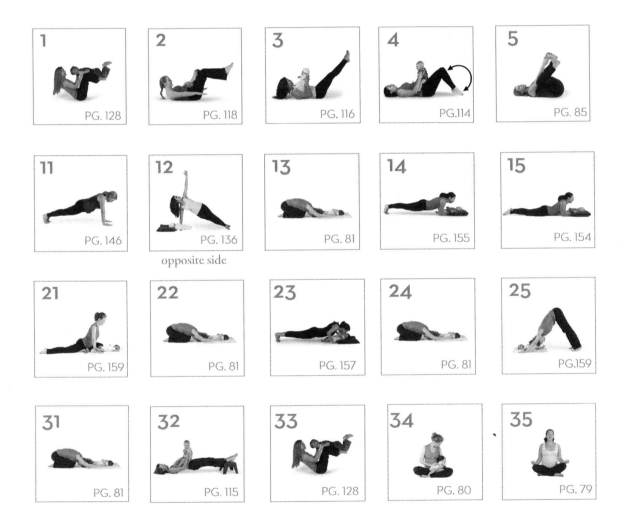

1 — PG. 128
2 — PG. 118
3 — PG. 116
4 — PG. 114
5 — PG. 85

11 — PG. 146
12 — PG. 136   opposite side
13 — PG. 81
14 — PG. 155
15 — PG. 154

21 — PG. 159
22 — PG. 81
23 — PG. 157
24 — PG. 81
25 — PG. 159

31 — PG. 81
32 — PG. 115
33 — PG. 128
34 — PG. 80
35 — PG. 79

Note that the Side Plank and Flying Pigeon Flow exercises are presented to be performed on one side at a time, so that when they are repeated in the routine, they are to be done on the opposite side. Other exercises are repeated for the sake of working several reps into a session.

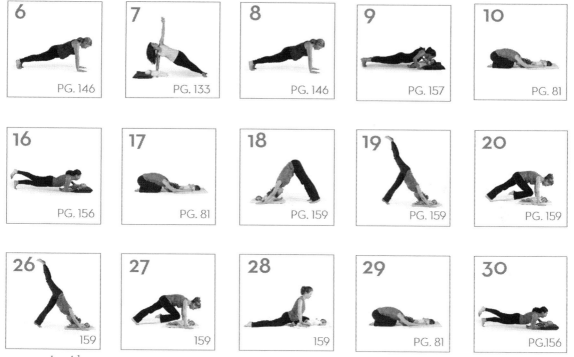

opposite side

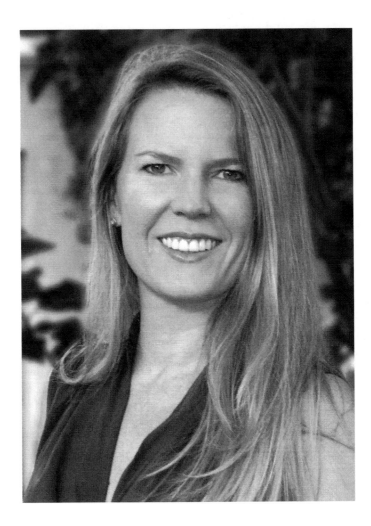

# About the Author

M<small>ICKY</small> M<small>ARIE</small> M<small>ORRISON</small>, P.T., ICPFE

Micky Marie Morrison is a licensed physical therapist with 15 years experience in women's health and pediatrics. As an International Childbirth Education Association certified perinatal fitness educator and mother of two, Micky began developing a progressive and intense prenatal and postpartum exercise program, first to meet her own needs, and later to meet those of her clients. CoreMama™ was born.

Micky's work with the CoreMama™ program demonstrated that women craved more of a challenge than what was typically offered in prenatal and postpartum programs. The new mothers and moms-to-be in the CoreMama™ classes were also inquisitive about proper nutrition and the changes in their bodies during and after pregnancy. Micky recognized the need for a comprehensive prenatal and postpartum fitness plan that would include all aspects of health and nutrition. *Baby Weight* was born.

Micky divides her time between La Antigua Guatemala, where she owns Healing Hands Therapy Spa, and South Florida, where she teaches the CoreMama™ program to new and expectant mothers, as well as to other healthcare and fitness professionals.

Made in the USA
San Bernardino, CA
27 February 2017